To Judy with hopes enjoy these tales.

12 Dec 94

Tales From My Little Black Bag

A Family Doctor's Memoir

John R. Ibberson M.D., C.M., F.C.F.P.

Detselig Enterprises Ltd.

Calgary, Alberta, Canada

Tales From My Little Black Bag

Canadian Cataloguing in Publication Data

Ibberson, John R. (John Rawcliffe), 1919-
Tales from my little black bag

ISBN 1-55059-093-6

1. Ibberson, John R. (John Rawcliffe), 1919-   2. Physicians
(General practice)--Canada--Biography.   I. Title.
R464.I22A3 1994   610'.92   C94-910933-9

© *1994 Detselig Enterprises Ltd.*
210-1220 Kensington Rd. N.W.
Calgary, Alberta, Canada
T2N 3P5

Detselig Enterprises Ltd. appreciates the financial support for our 1994
publishing program, from the Department of Canadian Heritage, Canada
Council and the Alberta Foundation for the Arts (a beneficiary of the
Lottery Fund of the Government of Alberta).

Edited by Linda Berry

Cover Design by Dean MacDonald

Printed in Canada   ISBN 1-55059-093-6   SAN 115-0324

Preamble

Some names and locations have been changed to protect peoples' identities. The author does not wish to cause embarrassment, nor find fault. This is a story as recalled from his point of view.

Dedication

To my supportive wife Ruth and our children, Bill, John and Nancy, who cared and encouraged me in all my careers.

Acknowledgements

My sincere appreciation to Jack Donoghue for his encouragement, instruction and editing without which this manuscript would have perished. To my son John for his initial editing of part I and to Ruth for the clarity of her suggestions; and to my sister-in-law, Betty Moilliett, who with Ruth helped me recall and write many of the events. To my niece, Mrs. Mary Miller for her editorial skills and her challenge to make me write deeper.

Contents

CHAPTER I

Inspirations

My best friend, David Forrester, died of leukaemia when I was seven years old. I did not understand his death; the last time I saw him was when our class walked past his open coffin at his funeral. Everyone said the doctors could do nothing to cure him, there was no cure. That made me sad and angry, as we were good friends and did everything together. Ultimately, David's death was a motivating factor in my decision to pursue a medical career.

My dream of becoming a doctor started in grade seven. A friend of my father, Dr. T.J. Gray, an ear, nose and throat specialist, who before specializing had been a country practitioner, returned to Humbolt, Saskatchewan during the Depression to collect past due accounts. On one occasion I was invited to go along as company. I don't recall whether we collected any accounts. I do remember the many stories with which Dr. Gray entertained me. This ignited my interest and from that day, I knew I wanted to be a doctor.

In Saskatoon we lived close to the City Hospital where I had a job throughout high school. Initially, I was an orderly, then moved to positions in x-ray and pharmacy. By the time I applied for admission to University, I had a clear idea of what medicine had to offer.

The day I received my university acceptance letter I remember talking with a senior surgeon, Dr. George Peterson. I clearly recall his comment.

"Well young fellow, I'll tell you what you will get out of medicine. You will always have a job, you will get enough to eat, you will have a bed on which you can sleep occasionally and you will never be bored. If you want more than that, do something else for a living."

He was correct! It has been satisfying. There have been times of fatigue extending to exhaustion, times of frustration and feelings of inadequacy, but I have never wanted to do anything else.

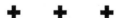

I spent my first three years of university at the University of Saskatchewan, majoring in pre-med for which I obtained a B.A. The university did not have a medical school then, but the Dean had made arrangements for the transfer of the top sixteen students to medical schools in other Canadian universities. I was accepted into second year medicine at Queen's University in Kingston, Ontario.

Eastern Canada was an eye-opener to me, a prairie kid accustomed to the large flat fields measured in quarter sections (160 acres); their farms were lilliputian in comparison. I couldn't imagine even turning a tractor around in their fields, let alone a combine or large thresher. They talked of fields in acres, I was accustomed to a small field being at least a quarter section. I could recall helping patients of my dad's at harvest time, riding a binder around a section of land: one mile by one mile square. When I first saw the eastern fields, I did not know how they could grow a worthwhile crop and make a living.

In finding a rooming house, fortune shone upon me. I moved into a third floor attic room in a house run by three maiden sisters, retired school teachers, who did their best to make us comfortable. The other two attic rooms held a classmate in in the same year of medicine and an engineering student. The second floor spare bedroom held another classmate in medicine.

The attic rooms were quite small, each with a single window and an outside wall which rose part way before sloping towards the ceiling. There was room enough for a desk, bookcase, bed and chest of drawers, a trunk and a wall closet. For one person it was adequate and cosy.

The house was a typical three story eastern brick home within walking distance of the university. These homes provided most of the residential accommodation for male students and most of us ate at the student's union building. There were some university residences for female students. In those days, I regret to say, Queen's did not take female students into medicine, so our classes were entirely male. Our professors demanded that we dress in a professional manner and show the utmost respect for patients and pathological specimens.

Don Beckett, an engineering student, occupied the back attic room. Ted Cameron, my good friend from Ottawa, who was in the same year of medicine, lived in the other front attic room. The second floor bedroom was rented by Jack McCarley from Vancouver, also in second year medicine.

We were a serious crew set on achieving our goals, but not without some fun. Jack was the most serious, a loner, who had a special girl friend. They married before we graduated and Jack continued his studies as they lived in an apartment. The second floor room was then taken by Jim Loynes, also in our medical class. We were equally poor and had similar methods of studying, summarize and constantly review. We could discuss problems and help each other understand and we each had a sense of humor which held us together. Not surprisingly, our marks were close, usually in the top third of the class. It was a good mutual support system.

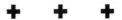

We had diverse summertime work to support our budding careers in medicine. Ted Cameron worked for Heinz in the quality control laboratory in Leamington, Ontario. Not surprisingly, he seldom ate ketchup during the rest of the year; he said he saw enough ketchup at work to last him a lifetime. Jack McCarley returned to North Vancouver to work with his father, a physician. Jim Loynes had many different jobs in the Toronto area. Don Beckett went to some large construction site and I went to the mountains to drive cars, trucks and buses for Jasper Park Lodge in Jasper, Alberta.

While at the University of Saskatchewan, I had started working at Jasper Park Lodge, first as a caddy, then as a driver. Our boss, a Scot named Mr. McDunnough, was a C.N.R. district passenger agent based in Winnipeg, who spent his summers handling tours for Jasper Park Lodge. He was a bachelor, superficially gruff but with a mellow core and a keen sense of business. In those days the C.N.R. sold tour packages which included a stay at Jasper Park Lodge, trips to the surrounding mountain spots and tours to the Columbia Icefields.

Many of the private guests, in comparison to the tour guests, reserved private cabins at Jasper Park Lodge for longer periods and played golf or toured in our hired limousines. We loved those private trips and did everything we could to earn a sizeable tip.

Our vehicles were Roadmaster Buicks, soft tops, four door convertibles with an additional windshield for back seat passengers. These were luxurious automobiles, ideal for sightseeing in the Rocky Mountains. When we were lucky enough to get a trip through to Lake Louise or Banff, we arranged to get a picnic lunch supplied by the chef and we stopped somewhere along the way. We all had our favorite spots. This, coupled with an encyclopedic memory of local history, fur trading stories, mountain names and animal antics, usually earned us a sizeable tip.

Our other vehicles were the big buses. As a senior driver I drove the "Icefields Bus." At 10 a.m., we picked up a full load at the Jasper Park Lodge entrance and, with appropriate stops at various streams and cascading falls and special view-points, we made our way to the Columbia Icefields, arriving at noon. The lunch time layover was two hours leaving lots of time for the tourists to see the Icefields, have lunch and buy souvenirs. Brewster and Rocky Mountain Tour bus loads came up from Banff and Lake Louise. After lunch I took their passengers heading for Jasper and they took my passengers heading for Lake Louise or Banff; thus each bus and driver returned to their own garage at night.

In the late thirties and early forties, the roads were narrow, gravel rather than paved, with steep hills and many "switchbacks" (tight turns) on the corners. We had to back up in order to negotiate the corners in "two-goes." We often had the back of the bus hanging out in space! The wide paved roads and easy corners of today are pleasant driving and one can enjoy breathtaking scenery.

One afternoon returning from the Icefields with a full load – about forty-eight passengers and their luggage – my air brakes blew as I started down the first set of switchbacks. No brakes, not even a prayer! We had nothing!

I ordered everyone to stay in their seats. Even with down gearing through all the gears in the transmission and the separate set of gears in the differential I could barely slow our progress. With each corner we were spraying gravel into the ditch like a shower head. Fortunately no one was coming up the road because we were using every available inch!

Finally, after four switchbacks we were down to the level of the Athabasca River as it starts its journey from the Icefields. We limped cautiously back to Jasper Park Lodge aware that we had no stopping power other than down gearing. We reached the Lodge intact but two hours late. One female passenger was very vocal in her complaints to my boss, Mr. McDonnough.

After unloading the passengers and their luggage, I took my bus up to the garage for washing and repairs. I was in my room over the garage changing into my work clothes when the phone rang. It was Mr. McDonnough.

"Ibberson, get down to my office, immediately!"

"Yes, Sir," I said.

He was seated behind his big desk off the lobby of the old lodge. There was a scowl on his face and thunder in his voice. This was a Mr. McDunnough unknown to me. His comments were brief and to the point.

"Ibberson, I understand you blew your air brakes coming down the switchbacks leaving the Icefields and one of your passengers tore her stocking. Is that correct?"

There were icicles hanging in the air! I replied, "That is correct, sir."

The frigid atmosphere deepened. There was a long silence and then Mr. McDunnough replied, "Ibberson, you know we do not tolerate that type of behavior. You are fired. Dismissed!"

I was speechless, offended and a little scared. It was early in the season and I was dependent upon this job to get back to medical school. Had I not driven that big bus skilfully and got it down the mountain side without turning it over or taking it into the ditch? If I hadn't, she would have torn more than her darned stocking. Really, there had to be some justice, somewhere, somehow! As I got to my room the telephone rang. It was Mr. McDonnough.

"What are you doing?"

"I was just thinking about packing and getting out of here, since you fired me," I replied.

"Don't be daft, boy. Get down here to my office, on the double." He wasn't fooling. His big rumbling voice was back. I dropped the phone and ran all the way to his office. There he sat behind that big desk. He had a grin on his face and his familiar cigar sticking out the side of his mouth.

"Well, don't look so glum. I thought we pulled that off very well, don't you?" he said with a grin.

"What are you talking about?" I said, completely confused.

With an incredulous look, he said, "You didn't know what that was all about? You didn't see that half open door? I thought we pulled that off superbly. That vocal female passenger who tore her stocking was behind that partially open door. She insisted on my firing you because you raised your voice to her when you told the passengers to remain in their seats. Now, do you get it?"

I was still annoyed and said, "All I know is that I did a good job getting that bus down the mountain side without rolling it and getting the passengers back to the lodge intact and for that I lost my job. Now how do I get back to medical school with enough money to pay for next year?"

He smiled and said, "You really are ticked off! You did a superb job getting that bus down the mountain side without rolling it. She doesn't realize how lucky she was to have a cool experienced driver. She is annoyed because she tore her stocking. The customer is always right, so I agreed to fire you and thought we put on a good act. What she doesn't know is that I didn't promise not to re-hire you. Now quit feeling sorry for yourself and quit wasting my time. Get back to work!"

I was learning about handling people and the basic skills of management. That summer job was excellent training. Little did I know how valuable that would be later in medical practice.

Mr. McDonnough was at heart an incurable romantic. He was a big man who wore a cowboy hat which allowed him to stand out in a crowd, the more easily to be identified in meeting his crowd of tour groups coming off the train. Both the C.N.R. and C.P.R. railways offered tours to large groups to see the Canadian Rockies. At that time the tours concentrated on Canadians and Americans since the war was threatening. Mr. McDunnough liked to hire legal and medical students to drive since they were in university for longer periods of time and could spend more summers on his staff. Proof of his romanticism and generosity was supported by his personally paying for accommodation at Jasper Park Lodge for any newlyweds from his staff. He covered his generosity with bluster and profanity which was ignored by the staff and the grateful newlyweds. On our wages, we could not afford the Lodge prices. The only way we could enjoy the amenities and scenery of Jasper Park was to work as staff.

Driving the four-door Buick "rag tops" did not pay as large a salary as driving the buses, but the opportunity for tips was greater. We all developed "tip generating" techniques. Lodge guests appreciated a running commentary based on historical knowledge of early explorers, the fur traders, the Indians and local characters. This involved self education, reading history books, government tourist information and on occasion, when lost, a superb imagination. One never let the facts destroy what could be made into a good story. We knew the names of all the mountains, valleys, rivers and streams and most of the animals and their habitats.

We improvised when we lacked knowledge. Those little mountain creatures – marmots – we re-christened "side-hole gougers" and told people facetiously that their legs were shorter on one side than the other because they always went around the mountain in one direction. "Watch closely to see if you can pick that up." It seemed the more inventive the story, the better the tip. Some days the animals would be on our side and they would act out the fanciful tale.

One afternoon, with a full bus load of passengers, I eased to a stop on the shores of Lake Edith, a small lake with a sandy shore. A large mother black bear was playing on the shore with her two cubs. As we stopped, she thought a retreat into the water was wise. With her nose she nudged one cub into the lake. The other cub was uncooperative, curious about other things and then downright resistant. He had other ideas. With almost the speed of light the mother's paw flashed through the air and a black ball of fur landed with a splash at least forty feet from shore. Discipline obviously varies little from animals to humans. That demonstration produced generous tips. Too bad I could not repeat the scenario!

Occasionally on the "Icefields run," we would arrange a free trip for one of the waitresses or chambermaids on their day off. They would sit in a front seat with instructions to be the first person off the bus and to offer a $5 tip with gratitude for an interesting trip. "Hold the bill up so other passengers can see it is a five-spot!" It was our $5 which was used to prime the pump.

Mrs. Baker, of the American chocolate firm, came to the same cabin for a month each summer. She was a motherly type and brought her grandchildren. Often I would drive her to church or to shop and arrange sightseeing side trips. She treated us as her sons and we reciprocated by treating her accordingly. I know she quietly helped some students complete their degrees.

Summers spent working in Jasper were an ideal variant from long months of intense study and we were working with people, ideal training for our future professional lives.

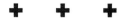

Early in our third year of medicine, my friend Ted Cameron and I were seized with concern about the war and attempted to enlist in the R.C.A.F. through the recruiting office in downtown Kingston.

The recruiting officer was more observant than we realized. He asked about our education and we both gave an incomplete answer, saying we had senior matriculation. Age-wise we were about five years beyond that qualification. The officer asked what we had been doing and we fabricated a story. Then he grabbed our hands to see if we had any work calluses – negative. Then he tricked us by saying, "Obviously, you fellows flunked out of university!" This was more than our pride could stand. We blurted out the truth of being part way through third year medicine with good marks.

As he called the Sergeant to throw us out, he made sense of the rejection by saying, "Yes, we need pilots – but we also need medical officers. By the time we get you trained as pilots you will almost be doctors, so don't waste my time. Stick with your original plans, we need you as Squadron M.O.s." His wisdom kept us on track.

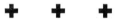

When we finished our third year at Queen's in the spring of 1942, rumors suggested we would be attending university non-stop until graduation. If true, we envisioned a financial crisis: we needed summer earnings to support winter tuition and room and board. I was selected by the class to speak to the Dean, Dr. Spencer-Melvin, a retired Army Medical Officer and our professor of physiology. There was no point in being oblique.

"Sir, we have heard rumors and the class has sent me to get facts."

"Quite so, Ibberson," he said, "you will all be attending university full time, without a break until graduation." He paused, "Your economic concerns have been anticipated. You will all be enlisting in the army tomorrow, with the rank of private." There was more. "The army will supply your uniforms, socks, boots, caps and great coats. There will be an allowance for quarters and rations." He easily slipped back into army parlance.

The following day we were enlisted, issued uniforms and assigned a sergeant. He tried to arrange parades and instruction but we were always busy in the hospital or on call for maternity or observers in the operating room or emergency room. Strangely, however, we always had time for pay-parade every Friday at noon. He was older and wise to the ways of youth and time had given him tolerance.

Most of us were better off financially. We had been going to university on a tight budget of about $50 per month for food and lodging, leaving about $5 per month for entertainment, namely dates. We now had $75 per month and our clothing and boots were issued by the army. The part time jobs disappeared. For most it was slinging beer in the pubs, for me it was part-time trips driving huge trucks hauling freight on the highways.

We had a few weeks off before we returned to university to start our fourth, fifth and final sixth year on a non-stop schedule. Jim Sinkins and I went separately to Peterborough to "intern" though we were only third year medical students. He worked in the lab at St. Joseph's Hospital and I worked in the lab, pharmacy and x-ray at the Civic Hospital. We both had some hair-raising experiences, all due to our lack of knowledge and experience and caused by our self-imposed importance; nothing serious but thought-provoking incidents.

One night I had to do an emergency white blood count on a young teenager, admitted with the tentative diagnosis of acute appendicitis. The attending surgeon said, in an effort to be helpful, that if the white blood count was over 14 000 he would operate that night. If the count was less, he would wait until morning, then re-assess the patient. I had technically been off duty and had a drink at one of the nurse's apartments during dinner. I was called back to do the white count as the person on duty was sick. I did not anticipate a problem. The first count came out at 14 000. The little white blood cells did not want to stay still within the microscopic counting chamber under the microscope. The second count was 13 800. I re-counted and resolved never to drink again. The third count was 14 000 even. The fourth count was 13 500. I had insufficient experience to realize that other factors would be involved in the surgeon making a decision to operate that evening. I was junior enough to think the entire matter rested upon the results of my white blood count.

I called the surgeon and told him my sorrowful story. He let me sweat a little, commiserated and said he would re-assess the patient's condition in the morning. I had a sleepless night, not knowing enough about the clinical picture to realize there was little danger of this child rupturing his appendix.

This made an impression upon me. Alcohol and work do not mix, ever!

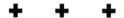

We returned to school and worked our way through three years of university in two years. Often we were the only students on campus, it was great as we had the pool and the Student's Union cafeteria to ourselves. We needed no sympathy. We had one day off for each of Christmas and New Year's Day! It did not occur to us that the professors and clinicians were also working daily to rapidly get us through to graduation in May, 1944. I don't think we complained any more than any other students. If we did, it didn't matter. No one listened, as they were busy with the war effort. The army needed medical officers, but first we had to intern for a year.

CHAPTER II
No Life Like It

My internship at the Vancouver General Hospital (V.G.H.) started on Gynaecology. This was a twenty-eight bed ward with a few private rooms, in the old traditional plan of hospitals. It was run by two extremely capable and efficient nurses. They may have been only a few years older than me but they were all business. "If you want to learn, we will teach you, if you want to be lazy we will make your life unbearable." They were good teachers. They presumed that I knew nothing and started at the beginning. I am forever grateful for lessons they taught me, lessons I have used daily throughout my life. We were short-handed, running that 1200 bed hospital with nine interns who often had to cover several services (departments) at once. During one holiday weekend, I was particularly busy and I recall going to the switchboard to look at the call schedule only to learn that I was the only intern on duty for the entire hospital!

The next month I was on Internal Medicine, then Psychiatry, then Urology; each month you moved to a new service. Being impatient, I enjoyed the surgical services more than the medical wards. I like to see an answer to problems quickly, rather than waiting weeks or months. Promotion came quickly; I was a junior intern for several months, then a senior and ultimately a resident. The pay started at $10.00 per month with board and room and laundry (during internship we were not paid by the army). With each promotion the pay increased by $5.00 per month. You worked at least ninety-two hours per week, often more since you were on call for a full twenty-four hours at a time. My wife says that I can lie down for ten minutes and sleep for nine and a half, a skill I learned as an intern. You worked and grabbed something to eat and slept when you could. It was an exciting life, what I had dreamed of. One soon forgot the fatigue. When you had a night off, you didn't spend it sleeping, you invited one of the nurses out!

I enjoyed working Emergency and spent several months there. Vancouver being a seaport town, you saw everything imaginable and some things beyond imagination. We were not supposed to ride the ambulances, but we did. I have been places in Chinatown where only as an intern were you safe. They knew you didn't have any money and you were there to help someone. We usually carried a heavy wrench in our back pocket, as insurance.

One night we got a call from the look-out on the Lions Gate Bridge, saying a boat coming in had signalled they needed to be met by an ambulance and doctor. We roared out into the pitch black night down to the docks and as the ship was berthing I hollered up to the Captain, "What is the emergency?" His answer was not what I expected. "We have an additional passenger we didn't start with!" I rushed on board and found the mother in the Captain's cabin with her newborn son still attached to the umbilical cord. I had nothing with which to tie the cord, so I cut it long and used my shoe lace as a tie. We could shorten the cord later under more sterile conditions. I'm quite sure the hospital never replaced that shoe lace. Both mother and babe did well, no infection and no problems.

Emergency was always busy. One night we were so crowded that all the beds and chairs were full. There was no space left when the ambulance brought in a semi-conscious drunk. The only space I could think of was the old bath tub in the washroom, "Put him there," I said. "I'll get to him later when we've relieved the congestion."

The truth is, I forgot about the patient until about 4 a.m. – then I asked one of the student nurses to check and see how he was. There was an arresting scream from the old washroom. We all rushed in; he was sound asleep in the tub, peaceful as could be. His toupee had slipped off his head and the ambulance boys had shoved it into his coat jacket breast pocket. Our conscientious student nurse thought the toupee was a rat on his jacket. He was oblivious to the turmoil, sleeping the sleep of the intoxicated. He had found a dry, warm spot and didn't intend it to go to waste. We woke him in time for breakfast, then discharged him, knowing he would be back, one of our chronic patients.

One evening, a mother came off the street-car with her three and a half year old son, a brown paper bag firmly pulled down to his ears. He did not appear to be in any obvious discomfort. Why the brown bag over his head? Once inside the emergency, with the admitting paper work done, we removed the bag. His head was firmly wedged, to ear level, in what used to be called a "thunder mug," an under the bed toilet pot. To slip the mug off seemed a simple task.

I used every trick I could think of and the mug remained unmoved! I tried lubricants, no go. Warmed oils, no go. Tugging, pulling, hitting with a rubber percussion hammer, no go.

In desperation I went to the engineering maintenance department for a small sledge hammer and a cold chisel. With the child firmly held on the operating room table by two nurses and me now enthusiastically hitting the cold chisel with the sledge hammer, we worked our way around the edge of the pot which flew off his head with a sucking sound and clattered on the tile floor with a startling crash.

The child seemed unconcerned, however I was sweating and the nurses were a little dishevelled. No, I didn't ask him why he put it there, in emergency you learn to not ask questions for which there is no logical answer.

Nightly we had stabbing and fight injuries, all a part of the life led by our clientele, the hookers, the muggers, the drug trade and people who did not limit their arguments to rational discussion, but rather to closed fists after a few beers. We also had the ordinary citizens with routine accidents.

When we were busy, which was most of the time, I had the habit of recording cases by drawing a picture of the affected part and indicating by a line where sutures were inserted and recording the number.

Early one morning, a young man came in with a bleeding foreskin torn at the back wherein there is a small artery. It was bleeding profusely. He wanted a band-aid and I told him it would not control the bleeding and we would have to use a little local anesthetic and put in a couple of sutures. That would fix the problem. He looked at me, visibly paled, clutched his private parts and said, "Stitches down there! Never. Just put on a bandage." I assured him it would not stay nor control the bleeding. He was most definite – a bandage only.

He was back in about an hour, blood all over. We injected the anesthetic and inserted two sutures which controlled the bleeding artery and he was fine. It became a busy night. Unthinkingly I drew a picture of what I had done and got on with thirty more cases.

During the 7 a.m. nurses shift change report, I heard the nurses giggling and paid no attention. The head-nurse, Miss Phyllis Neal, was a cracker-jack professional. When asked what that was all about, she tossed her head, put on her dignity and commented, "It is nice to know it isn't always the woman who pays!" We did not discuss it further.

Some doctors are adept at working emergency and enjoy it, others don't. You learn to work under pressure, to think quickly and adapt, so that it becomes a reflex. I loved emergency because of the variety and crazy things that happened. Every doctor who has worked emergency has hundreds of stories, all true. These are but a sampling.

When I was promoted to being a resident on Orthopaedic Surgery, I encountered the "Chief," Dr. Jack Naden. He was a typical orthopod, quick, untiring, demanding, a good surgeon, not very tall in stature but with a monumental ego, full of confidence. In fact, he was almost as good as he thought he was. He never said please or thank you and he expected your best at all times. It was good training.

We were busy, the war was on and all the young orthopaedic surgeons were in the services. We started to operate at 7 a.m. and did not stop for coffee, cigarettes or lunch until we were done, often about four in the afternoon. Then it was time to hit the wards.

Dr. Naden had 160 beds in V.G.H. and I would see all the patients, write orders, write histories longhand (there were no facilities for interns to dictate histories or reports as there are today), change casts, select instruments for the next day's surgery, see the cases in emergency for admission and review the x-rays. He would go to his office and keep a nurse and two secretaries busy seeing about 80 patients and get home about 10 p.m. It was good training for running a busy practice and office, in later years.

From him, I learned the following technique: if I suggested we handle a patient's problem by doing "so and so," he would solve the problem by any other method. If I approached the solution obliquely and said, "You know that patient we have with the XYZ problem. I have been thinking about what you suggested (this would be the first we had ever talked about it). When you said we should do so and so, I have been thinking about that method and I think it will work." He would show no surprise, but reply, "If you think that will work Ibb, why don't you do it that way. Book the case at the end of today's list and you do it." He was enough of an egotist that it had to be his idea. Of course most of my ideas came from him – he was doing the teaching. Once I figured out the system, we got along fine. I have since used this oblique approach on similar people.

A disease which kept us busy is seldom seen today, thank goodness, because the deformity and consequences it caused were severe. Osteomyelitis is an infection in the bone causing abscesses within the cancellous or spongy part of the bone. As a consequence, we had to approach the long bones in the arms and legs with equally long incisions to remove a portion of the hard bone to allow the pus to drain from the soft cancellous bone. This caused terrible scars but saved the limb from amputation. The discovery and use of penicillin and subsequent antibiotics has all but eliminated osteomyelitis. During the war, when penicillin was discovered and initially used, many legs and arms were saved from amputation because the osteomyelitis caused by open dirty gunshot wounds was successfully treated.

We had been busy for months and I needed the weekend off. Furthermore, I had met a smashing redhead working in pediatrics. I started my campaign on Tuesday, pointing out stories I had heard of the great salmon fishing across the channel at Campbell River. How long it had been since Dr. Naden had taken his sons fishing. The next day comments about his fatigue and his need for a few days off. Bingo, by Friday he announced he was taking the boys fishing at Campbell River and he had even chartered a flight for this short hop.

It looked like I might get the weekend off. He phoned from the airport Saturday morning, "Ibb, since you are going to have a slack weekend, would you mind slipping down to the chronic hospitals Glen and

Grandview and look at some of the chronic cases we have and change any casts that need fixing. And oh yes, there are some bone films they have been asking us to read over in the T.B. wing. Could you do that also?"

The week-end was deteriorating. What with body casts to change, emergency fractures to see, a stack of films in the T.B. wing that was five feet tall, I never had time for my date with the red head!

Part way through our first case Monday morning, I remember it was a back fusion, Dr. N. asked how my date went. I was flabbergasted; I had said nothing!

"You kept me so busy we never went out on a date."

He chuckled as he said, "She's not your type."

"How do you know what my type is anyway?"

"You can't get away with anything," was his know-it-all reply. Sometime later the red head and I went out on a date, and I guess he was right because nothing came of it.

Maternity was a busy and interesting rotation. Dr. Herb MacGregor had taken his discharge from the R.C.A.F. and returned to V.G.H. to refresh his obstetrical skills before returning to assist his father in practice in Penticton. We were a great pair; we ran that separate obstetrical hospital in the V.G.H. complex like a piece of well-oiled machinery. It was almost routine to do at least 12-14 deliveries in a twelve hour shift.

This was my first experience handling black patients. There had not been any black patients in my exposure to obstetrics in Saskatoon or Kingston. To me it was thought-provoking and prophetic to realize that they are born as white as the rest of us. The melanin in their skin darkens quickly, within forty-eight hours, when exposed to ultraviolet light. Why do some people have such violent reactions to skin color, when we all start the same? Maybe "The Man Upstairs" is trying to tell us something. Are we listening?

We learned a lot of obstetrics and gynaecology in a short period of time, the joys and the tragedies. I can still recall a beautiful eighteen year old admitted after a "street" abortion during which her uterus was perforated. She was deathly sick with peritonitis, a massive infection of the abdominal cavity, caused by the perforation of her uterus. Antibiotics had not yet been discovered, only the precursor to the sulphanilamide group of drugs and it was ineffective. I watched that girl die of peritonitis over the period of a week. For reasons I cannot explain, I often think of that girl when I am shaving and the crushing guilt of the mother who sought a back room abortion rather that allow a birth out of wedlock.

While working emergency one night, the ambulance came roaring in and the boys said they had just picked up an M.I. (myocardial infraction, or heart attack). They wheeled the stretcher in and I got my first look at the patient – it was my father. Being the oldest child, I was close to my father; never closer than when our eyes met as he came in on the ambulance stretcher. His myocardial infarction was severe and he was in shock. My adrenalin started pumping and I issued orders automatically, starting an intravenous (I.V.) to gain access to the circulatory system, control the pain and get a cardiogram to assess the damage and the rhythm.

He had been at a Vancouver Dental Association dinner listening to his old friend Dr. John Clay of Calgary. Fortunately, in the next room of the Hotel Vancouver was a dinner meeting of Vancouver doctors. When he collapsed he was immediately attended to by a doctor, who recognized him. The physician knew I was interning at the V.G.H.

Once we had the immediate emergency controlled, we had a minute to talk before the sedation took over. He looked me in the eye and said, "This is a real bad one, isn't it?" I was full of bravado and said, "You've had bad ones before. The medication I gave you should start relieving the pain any minute now." He became very serious, looking me squarely in the eyes, "I'm sorry if this doesn't turn out well, your mother and sister will fall apart. You will have to look after them." His assessment was absolutely correct.

He died some hours later, in my arms. I cried. I knew we could not save him after my initial examination. He was my best friend. I still miss him.

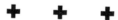

After completing internship, our lives as potential medical officers again came under army control. We were sent off to Camp Borden in Ontario where we spent the first eight weeks of officer training in the sand and wind; then a further four weeks at Brockville. All this with the rank of private. Fortune smiled upon me and gave me a bunk mate from the Veteran's Guard who had served in the 1914-18 war. He was originally a sergeant returning for officer training. He taught me tricks about how to keep a rifle bore shiny, how to prepare for dress parade and hundreds of secrets of coping with basic training. He was an old time survivor and I was a willing student.

We were supposed to be doctors, not infantry soldiers, but this was not so in the eyes of the army which believed one started at the bottom, learned the fundamentals, completed basic training and hoped to survive. The army believes you learn to take orders before you give them. With luck maybe you can work your way up the ranking scale. As with life, it is important to learn the business before you start running it. We graduated as second lieutenants.

My base posting was Vancouver, Military District XI. Although I arrived shortly after VE day, June 1945, we still had to deal with the Pacific Theatre of war. One of my early assignments was to go to Quebec City and travel west with a Troop Train carrying soldiers returning from the U.K. for discharge. All our passengers were from Military Districts X and XI, Winnipeg and west. They were a combination of "Well" and "Walking Wounded." The "Well" were entitled to one month's pre-discharge leave before returning for their final medical examination and discharge from the army. The walking wounded were assessed and admitted to the Veterans' Hospital closest to their home where they continued treatment until healed. Then they received their final medical examination and discharge from the army.

One of our community health concerns was venereal disease and preventing or controlling its further spread. To me it made no sense to allow these men one month's leave and then have them return for an examination and blood test for syphilis as part of their discharge medical. My plan was to take blood samples on the train between Quebec City and Ottawa, then ask the lab to telegraph the names or numbers of the positive results to me on the train. This way, the men could be diverted for treatment before taking the infection home.

This was a deviation from policy, a major decision for the army. My Colonel thought the idea had merit, but it got shot down further up the chain of command. Evidently I did not have sufficient rank to be considered capable of original thought. That is the way the army worked then.

For my trip, since this had never been done before, I was advised to draw from stores a number of Pannier Kits. When I looked at these kits, there were enough wooden splints to build a house. I elected to take my little black bag to the dispensary and advise the pharmacy sergeant to go for coffee, on the understanding that I would leave him a list of items taken. My judgement failed to include two items. I did not anticipate these fellows hanging out the windows of these old railway coaches looking at scenery – they couldn't get enough of it. Unfortunately, they got cinders in their eyes, from the coal burning locomotives. Secondly, they ate and ate – we could barely keep up to their appetites for eggs, milk and cheese, nor the resulting constipation. I corrected my pharmaceutical deficit by buying what I needed, anesthetic eye ointment and a large bottle of cascara, in a small drug store when we stopped to take on water for the locomotive. The recommendation went into my report for a properly equipped bag. Incidentally, I had no use for the splints.

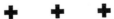

After a few trips, I was posted to Little Mountain Camp, located in what is now Queen Elizabeth Park, Vancouver. I should have bought property, but at that time I had no insight, nor money. Within a short time I was promoted to the rank of Captain and became the senior medical officer, running the sick bay with my own staff of non-commissioned officers and nursing sisters. We had all the usual treatment facilities and a ten bed ward. All the medical officers on staff were extremely busy doing discharge medical examinations.

Several incidents come to mind. My venereal disease control officer was a superb doctor doing a job he hated. Weekly he would come to my office to say he was quitting. I would point out that he had no such option, quoting from the King's Rules and Regulations, then I would take him to the Officers' Mess, buy him a drink or two and screw up his courage for another week. One week he came to my office with a different look in his eye.

"See that big fellow in the treatment room," he said. "He just came in and put his 'business' on the table and said, 'Doc, can you fix it up for Saturday night?' I don't have to put with such nonsense. I'm not a mechanic! I don't care what the King says in his Rules and Regulations. I quit!"

I knew he was serious. "Well Dave," I replied, "Maybe there is a post graduate course where I can send you for a break."

The only course available at that time was in Psychiatry, at the Veterans' Shaughnessy Hospital.

Today, this delightful man is a much respected psychiatrist practicing in the West. Maybe I had something to do with redirecting his life. Maybe anything was better than being a V.D. Control Officer, even becoming a shrink.

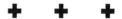

Several weeks later, my senior Nursing Sister came to my office seeking orders for a Captain in the Medical Corps, we had nicknamed Shirker.

"I don't understand your request Sister" I said.

She told me that he had said, on my orders, after lunch he was to lie down for several hours!

"To use a bed in the sick bay, sir, I need a written order," she said.

At this point, one of my medical officer friends overheard this conversation and his eyebrows went skyward. We were extremely busy and one of my officers was pulling a juvenile stunt like this. My patience was stretched to its limit and I reacted by saying to my Nursing Sister:

"Sister, please prepare a 2cc syringe with a 20 gauge 2 1/2 inch needle and fill it with denatured alcohol. Captain Sinclair and I will be down immediately to give the intramuscular injection." I then said to Jack Sinclair, "You whip back the blankets and I'll let him have it in the rear."

Alcohol stings fiercely when injected into a muscle. He was back to work immediately; limping, but back to work.

That evening he came to my office to request a transfer. Not surprisingly, the transfer orders and transport tickets were already prepared and lying on my desk. I signed the order and never saw him again, nor wanted to.

The next day, Captain Sinclair said, "You don't suppose that injection will cause the skin to slough?" I'm afraid I was completely devoid of compassion.

"I don't know," I said, "and I don't particularly care. If it does, he will have scar as a reminder." Possibly this was a poor outlook on my part, but I was fed up with his childish behavior.

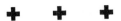

My means of transport was a big Harley Davidson 80 motorcycle. It was an ex-Vancouver police bike which I acquired when I was an intern. It was a silver colored brute, the largest bike they made. It still had a hole in the front fender where the siren had been when it was an active police bike. One couldn't buy a car due to the war and gasoline was rationed. The bike provided fifty miles to the gallon of exciting wind blown transportation; however, as the miles piled up the spark plugs kept fouling, the oil lines leaked, the chain stretched and I couldn't get parts. One morning I came into my office complaining about the behavior of my bike. Soon Slim, my ambulance driver, came in with a request to borrow my bike to run some errands for the Staff Sergeant. I didn't ask, why don't you use the ambulance. I automatically said, "Sure, here are the keys. I won't need it until this evening."

That evening, when I went out to climb on my Harley, I noticed new fuel lines, new plugs and a new chain. It drove like a dream. The next morning I called Slim into my office and asked him where he had run errands for Staff Sergeant Cheverton. He said he had gone to a number of places, including the Royal Canadian Ordnance Corps (R.C.O.C) depot. They serviced dispatch rider's bikes. I told Slim what I had noticed about my bike.

"Did they have any bikes down there?"

"Yes sir, they did," he replied.

"You don't suppose a bike went into moth balls with a stretched chain and fouled plugs and leaking fuel lines, do you?"

"I don't know sir, I was only doing errands." Slim had been in the Army for a long time!

"Do you happen to know what the Sergeant drinks at the R.C.O.C. depot?"

"Rye sir, he drinks rye."

"If I were to call the officers' mess and request a bottle be put on my tab, could you see that it is delivered to the Sergeant with my thanks?"

"Yes I could, Sir. I'm sure he would be pleased."

I have always found it prudent to say thank you!

My Staff Sergeant Cheverton was largely responsible for my success. He was old enough to be my father, a veteran of WWI (I'm sure he lied about his age to enlist). He ran our establishment with great efficiency, and even though I was the officer in charge, I didn't interfere.

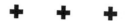

One evening Dr. Russ Neilson, one of my mentors in general surgery at the Vancouver General Hospital, called me at home. I was living with my widowed mother. Dr. Neilson wondered if I could get the morning off from the army and assist him at Infants' Hospital with a morning of harelip and cleft palate cases. His intern did not like working on tiny babies because he had forearms like salami sausages, and when he put his large arms on these tiny chests, the infants quit breathing. I assured Dr. Neilson that the army could carry on without me and I would be delighted to assist him with the morning's surgery.

He was a general surgeon who was interested in children's surgery and made a hobby of repairing harelips and palates. This was before the development of plastic surgery. He saved his cases and did them in batches outside of the croup (bronchitis) season. He preferred to do his harelips at six-to-twelve weeks of age; the cleft palates at a somewhat older age.

Infants' Hospital was technically a part of the large Vancouver General Hospital, but was situated on a separate site on Haro Street in the west end of Vancouver. They admitted children up to two years of age and were self contained with their own operating room, lab, x-ray and kitchen. Their instruments and anesthetic masks were small to meet the needs of their small patients. The total capacity was about 150 cribs.

At 7:30 a.m. the next morning, my ambulance driver delivered me to Infants'. I rushed up to the second floor which contained the surgical suite. There I encountered an official looking lady in her starched bib and apron uniform.

"I am Dr. Ibberson," I informed her. "I'm here to assist Dr. Neilson."

"Oh no, you're not," she said and disappeared into one of the adjacent sterilizing rooms.

I thought I was impressive in my uniform, wearing service ribbons above my left breast pocket and showing three pips of rank on my epaulets. I was speechless and quite taken aback.

After a minute she returned and said, "Look I'm sorry, if the intern scrubs we won't have enough sterile gowns for everyone. There is a war on, you know!" (Here I am in uniform). "We are short of supplies. The intern has to have a certain number of scrubs and he is booked for these cases."

"Pardon me," I said in annoyance. "Dr. Neilson called me last night and specifically asked me to assist him this morning." "I don't know anything about that," she said in a definite manner. "All I know is, the intern is booked to scrub. If you want to talk to him, I last saw him on the fourth floor. You two sort it out." She was quick to reply. With a swirl of her starched skirt she was gone, like quick silver.

I found the intern. He did not want to scrub, he had too many very sick babies to rescue that morning.

We started the morning's surgery, one case after another. I was aware that this "official" lady was in and out of the operating room taking these little patients back to their cribs, settling them and putting restraints on them so they could not disturb their dressings.

On our last case, she scrubbed in as the surgical nurse. It went smoothly. She handed a needle driver with suture and needle up to Dr. Neilson, he looked at it and said, "I thought I asked to have my sutures cut eleven inches long." No reply from the scrub nurse, she simply passed up a sterile ruler. We measured the suture – exactly eleven inches.

Who does she think she is, I said to myself? Just because she obviously runs this place smoothly and is the Matron, she isn't God! I should have known better.

We finished the case in record time. Instruments and sutures and anything else we needed came flying up to us, even before we knew we needed them. The responsibility for this surgery was clearly on our shoulders. There were no deficiencies in her operating room, nor her staff.

Infants' Hospital was special. It had its own dining room, linen table cloths and serviettes, china and cutlery. If they didn't ask you to stay for lunch, there was no other place to eat in the west end of Vancouver in those days. They were quite selective in their invitations. My priorities were to get back to my army duties, so I left.

This Matron lady returned from bedding down our last case and invited Dr. Neilson to stay for lunch; he was an old favorite of the staff. She then asked if Dr. Abrahamson or Robertson or whoever he was, meaning me, would stay.

Russ Neilson said, "You mean he made it. He got an invitation to stay for lunch the first time he is here? Wow! He had to go back to his army duties – he got an invitation to stay for lunch the first time! That must be some kind of a record."

The next day, I phoned Infants' and asked to speak to the Matron, Miss Marriott, who eventually came on the line.

"How would you like to go out to a show and dinner?" I asked. There was more than an appropriate pause, then, "Okay."

"When could you go?" I enquired. "Possibly tonight?"

"No," she replied.

"Tomorrow?"

"No."

"The next night?" I was getting desperate.

"No," she answered.

"Well then, what night?" I was in a quandary.

"I can't go until a week from next Thursday."

"My gosh, woman, I'm in the army. I could be posted anywhere by then!"

"I'm sorry, but that is the soonest I'm free," she said with some finality.

So we went out a week from next Thursday after ten days of anticipation.

After the show we were hungry so we drove to the original White Spot on South Granville for a turkey burger and boysenberry pie. I had changed into civilian clothes and somehow forgot to transfer all my money from my uniform. When the bill came, it was embarrassing as she had to use her "mad money" to pay for it. What a romantic start.

As Matron, she had her own suite and lived within the hospital. I suspect the hospital switchboard was overburdened with her social calls. I learned later that after I had taken her home at midnight, she had gone out with one of the interns. These women were liberated before the word had been invented. They had their own dining room and guests by invitation only; their own switchboard with calls screened before they came on the line; and their own quarters. If not liberated, they were certainly independent.

CHAPTER III
To the Bush and Back

When I got home from our first date there was a message from my Colonel: "I'm looking for a volunteer and since you have training in orthopaedic surgery, you have just volunteered. Be on the coastal streamer to Alert Bay. It leaves at 4 a.m. from Pier Number 4. You are taking over the operation of St. George's Hospital for the Columbia Coast Mission, on loan from the army for one month. They expect you."

When I arrived at Alert Bay, I wrote Miss Marriott a note saying that I had been posted and that was the reason I hadn't called as promised. I wasn't sure of her first name, hence the Miss Marriott. That note recently reappeared when I was getting something out of the Safety Deposit Box. I guess it was important to someone.

The situation at Alert Bay was unique. There was a clapboard building nestled on the hillside and facing the bay. Run by the Anglican Church, the Columbia Coast Mission served the needs of the surrounding Indians, loggers and fishermen. Their small steamer plied the camps in the many inlets along the inside passage between Vancouver Island and the mainland. Alert Bay itself is on a small island off the northern tip of Vancouver Island. The community boasted a fish cannery, logging offices, a general store, some engine repair shops and the B.C. police residence with holding cells. A large part of the island was an Indian Reservation.

When I arrived in November, 1945, it was raining and foggy, typical weather for the fall. No one at the hospital knew anything about me, nor where I was to stay. A great welcome! After much scurrying, I was settled into quarters in an annex to the hospital. I hate the word annex. It conjures up visions of something saggy and leaking hooked onto the side of a building, and this annex fit that description.

My first duty was to make rounds at the hospital. I found several cases of pneumonia and severe bronchitis, a couple of Indians recovering from acute alcoholism, some elderly patients and three loggers with fractured hips, the result of accidents. They were just lying there, no traction, no splinting, no fixation of their fractures – and these injuries were three weeks old! My orthopaedic instincts came to a boil. That was not good enough! There was an obvious lack of leadership and guidance. These Workmens' Compensation Board patients should have had some traction to stabilize their fractures. If active treatment was not available, they should have been stabilized and sent to where they could receive adequate treatment. I was upset and angry.

The next morning we started running that institution like a hospital, with objectives and priorities. My investigations revealed the Matron wished to retire, so we accommodated her with a replacement.

Assessing our facilities, we had a doctor's office with good examining rooms, an operating room, an x-ray, a lab, several wards and a well equipped kitchen and laundry. All the elements for success if one added some skills and hard work.

The fractured hip patients were x-rayed, supported on an apple box. A little intravenous anesthetic, insert three sterile surgical Kirschner wires, re-x-ray, then select the best positioned wire across the fracture site, pull out the other two wires, select the proper length of Smith-Petersen nail, a small skin incision, hammer in the S/P nail, re-x-ray to confirm position, a single skin suture and the job was done. I had done oodles of these cases for my chief in orthopaedics. Now these loggers had reduced stable fractures held in a good position; they could be up, but not weight bearing and were on their way to having a healed fracture in six to eight weeks. They did not need to be sent out. The equipment was there, though a little primitive; all that was needed was someone with the training and skills. No wonder my Colonel had volunteered me.

As winter passed, each day wet and foggy, new crises emerged, some funny, some routine and some alarming. Technically I was on loan to the Mission for one month. My salary was to be continued by the army at the rank of Captain, the Mission was to add a supplement to bring the remuneration to the equivalent of the rank of Major. Weeks passed, extending into the first month and I received no pay from either source. Rations and quarters were supplied by the hospital, but no pay and consequently no amenities.

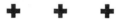

This was unsatisfactory. Discussions with the local hospital authorities generated excuses, not action. Letters to Army Headquarters disappeared into a void known as the mail. Radio contact at that distance and time of year was impossible. Here I was working hard, treating local residents, loggers, fishermen, Indians and receiving no income.

Although hired to provide medical services, I had been exposed to some dental training, my father having been an oral surgeon. The only person who extracted teeth was the engineer on the Columbia Coast Mission steamer. He used a combination of pliers and mechanical tools of his trade, but no anesthetic.

The market was there. I had local anesthetic and training in how to use it. Scrounging through the hospital cupboards, I found some dental forceps and other basic instruments. With necessity at hand, inevitably a new entrepreneur was born.

Since I used local anesthetic and he didn't and since our charges were identical, fifty cents a tooth, and I could control the bleeding and prescribe medication for pain, my dental practice flourished. George, the engineer, did not mind being relieved of the pesky dental emergencies. A source of income was created, amenities followed.

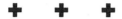

It was cold and foggy, a light drizzle had been falling for two days. There was not much activity on the island, because everyone was trying to stay dry and warm. My hospital office phone rang and it was Sergeant Bill Davidson of the local B.C. police force with an invitation.

"Doc, how would you like to go fishing?" he said. "Don't forget to bring your little black bag."

That should have made me suspicious, but I was such a neophyte. Sergeant Davidson was one of the few people who helped maintain my sanity in this gloomy place. He guided me through many adventures which he called learning experiences. This was no exception. He never went fishing from the police boat, but my nature is not one of suspicion. Once he was sure we were too far from shore to swim back, he gave me the rest of the story, which had nothing to do with fishing.

Sergeant Bill had received a panic radio call from one of the small logging camps. One of the loggers, a big Swede, was standing in a clearing at the camp swinging his razor sharp double-bladed felling axe and no one could get closer than fifteen feet. The police were supposed to do something about it and I was the volunteer. As in so many emergencies, the crucial details so desperately needed were not at hand, so we could only speculate.

After chugging up the inlet for about an hour, we arrived at the camp. They welcomed us with enthusiasm, all talking at once. Making my way through the dockside group of loggers, I was aware of their tension and anxiety as we walked along the path to the camp. Standing in a clearing was our patient, Lars; a powerfully built Swede, six foot two with the athletic build of a man who cuts down gigantic trees for a living. His eyes were wide open with a maniacal look. He was standing alone, crying and pleading with everyone to stay away while swinging his axe around his head.

After looking at this fellow, from about fifteen feet, the diagnosis was clear; a manic-depressive in the manic phase. Our consultation was carried out by shouting, since safety required a buffer zone. As I asked questions, the diagnosis became even more obvious. His mental breakdown had been coming on for several weeks. Physical isolation in the logging camp and personal isolation caused by him having only rudimentary English skills had aggravated the situation. He had been unable to sleep for the previous four nights. This was not the routine insomnia that we all suffer occasionally, this was the wide awake, hyperactive manifestations of the manic phase of manic-depression, a serious mental illness.

The cause of manic-depression is unclear. Sometimes there is a family history but not often. We do not know what sent Lars off the deep end and his English skills were insufficient to obtain an in-depth history. No one spoke Swedish. In lay terms, the patient in the manic phase of a manic-depression goes faster and faster until they feel as if they will fall apart, and without treatment they figuratively do. In the depressed phase, they may become so withdrawn that they are unreachable and unresponsive to treatment.

This emergency demanded action; he had the axe, I had my little black bag which contained ampoules of sodium pentothal, a rapid-acting sedative often used intravenously for short lasting anesthetics. I could guarantee sleep. Lars had not slept in four days, 96 hours to be exact, and he was desperate. We were both dealing from a position of strength.

Before the entire camp, a deal was made. "Lars," I said, "I'm a doctor and I know what the problem is. I can guarantee you some sleep. Put down your axe and come into the bunk house. I have a special medicine that goes in your arm to put you to sleep. You haven't had any sleep in four nights, I know I can help you."

There was a long pause while he thought about what I had said. Maybe it had to undergo mental translation. Did he understand me? I had tried to use simple terms. After about 45 seconds, which seemed like 45 minutes, he gradually lowered the axe, then dropped it on the ground and slowly walked toward the bunk house. I followed.

The rest of the camp held back. To assume control of the situation, I had to be positive. As Lars dropped onto his lower bunk, I joined him and opened my little black bag to get what I needed; this was not the time for small talk. If anything, he was bigger lying on that bunk. His veins were like large pipes. I filled the syringe with pentothal, mentally calculating the dose for this giant. I slipped the needle into the vein and cautiously and slowly started the injection. He became more and more drowsy and soon drifted off into unconsciousness. The entire camp peering through the window and doorway burst into a cheer.

Now that he was immobile, I could attach an intravenous drip of 5% glucose and water to the same needle and maintain access to his blood stream and inject additional pentothal drug into the intravenous tubing as required. We were over the immediate crisis, now the real thinking could begin. We were miles from a sizeable hospital, let alone one with a psychiatric unit. The closest was Essondale Mental Hospital, New Westminster. Telephone connections were non-existent from the logging camp, however I was told the coastal supply boat would call the next day. Was it possible to keep this patient safely sedated that long? I had no other option. I wrote out a dosage schedule and left chloral hydrate, an inject-able sedative. This was to be used as an intra-muscular injection if necessary. We also rigged a modified restraining jacket, to be used only if required. We left Lars in the hands of his fellow workers, having done all we could at that point, and returned to Alert Bay.

With much difficulty, I eventually got through to Essondale Hospital to alert them of Lars' pending admission. I would like to report that he recovered, unfortunately he continued in a manic phase in spite of intensive treatment and died about a week after his admission to hospital.

This happened long before the discovery of the drug Lithium, which is almost a specific treatment for patients with this diagnosis. Most manic-depression patients today, with support therapy and Lithium med-ication, lead stable, normal lives. The biggest difficulty with these pa-tients is maintaining them on regular therapy. Even today, many patients with mental health and emotional problems, once they start feeling well, have a tendency to discontinue their medications and their symptoms return.

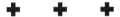

The Chief had been a magnificent specimen of West Coast Indian; tall, skin of bronze, rippling muscles, knowledgeable in forestry and fishing, a true leader of his people. Unfortunately, he was now aged, shrunken, wrinkled and fighting for each labored breath, a tragic terminal situation. He had been brought to the hospital in a semi-conscious state caused by a failing heart and kidneys, complicated by pneumonia. The outlook for his survival was grave.

Local customs demanded that if the Chief was apt to die, the band council members had to be there. Who they were or where they were or how to get them to the hospital in time, I had no idea. The only certain fact was that the chief was dying.

A call to my source of all things practical, Sgt. Bill Davidson, resulted in this peculiar conversation.

"Bill, this is the doctor. I have a problem. The old chief is in hospital dying of heart and kidney failure. He may die tonight and I don't know how to inform the band council."

"No problem," he answered, "I have the chief's brother in the cell downstairs. I'll turn him loose. He can round up the council members, then return to jail, lock himself in and throw the keys out onto the floor."

I was too busy to give this more than momentary thought, and shortly after, the Indians started arriving to pay their respects to the Chief.

Confirming my prognosis, the Chief died early the next morning, ending an era. The next morning, as I recalled that strange sequence of events, I purposely went to the police office for coffee.

"Bill," I said, "your scheme for rounding up the Indians worked fine, but why would the Chief's brother come back to jail, lock himself in and throw the keys out on the floor?"

Bill answered with a little impatience. "Simple, this is a small island and there is no place for him to go. In jail, eating my wife's good cooking combined with a dry place to sleep – he never had it so good!" He paused, "Why should I lose a night's sleep? He was there in the morning, wasn't he? He may be a petty criminal, but he is not stupid. You can't always do things by the book, Doc." Bit by bit, I was learning the ways of the practical world. I had interesting teachers.

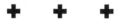

Old Joe Boggs was found dead in the woods by a passing Indian who informed the police, Sgt. Davidson. The remains were brought to the hospital for certification of death. At this point, as Coroner, I became involved.

After examining this broken body with a large depressed portion of skull, it was obvious that death had occurred due to an accident in felling a large tree.

I said to Sergeant Bill, "Obviously, this man has died as a result of being crushed by a falling tree."

"I know that," said Bill. "You have to certify his death and we have to call a Coroner's Inquest because it is an accidental death and we need to know how it happened. Up here you are the Coroner and as such you run the inquest. As the senior police official, I will call the necessary people to form a Coroner's Jury."

Great, I thought. I'm wearing four hats of authority, now I'm the coroner as well as the doctor, the dentist and the Public Health Officer. The principles of a coroner's inquest I knew, but I had never acted as a coroner nor run an inquest.

Sergeant Davidson knew all the rules and all the provincial legislation to form a Coroner's Jury and how to execute its purpose. The selected jury was made up of loggers, fishermen and storekeepers. The jury was a great collection of hard working, practical and down to earth people. I was impressed by one old logger dressed in a plaid Mackinaw jacket, toothless, inquisitive and chewing, or rather gumming, a plug of tobacco.

The jurors viewed the corpse and then listened to my extensive description of the type of head injury Joe had suffered. I had diagrams and drawings and sketches on the blackboard to explain how the injury had torn the tentorium of the brain and lacerated the cerebellum and the effect this had upon the vital functions of Joe's body and how such a state was incompatible with life. I did an excellent job of explaining basic physiology and trauma-induced death. I was quite proud of myself. I explained everything I had learned in six years of medical school and one year of internship. This was an exercise in superlative pathological teaching. My pride, however, was short lived.

Sergeant Bill said to the jurors, "Now you all know why you are here and why you were sworn in. We have called this inquest to clearly find out what killed Joe Boggs."

My toothless friend, the juror, gumming his plug, said, "Yah, I know why I'm here. Old Joe was a friend of mine. I heard what the Doc said, I'm not sure I understood all his big words; but the way I figure it, Joe was cutting down this great Jeezly cedar and the butt kicked back, hit him on the head, his brains spilled out on the ground and he croaked."

Jury dismissed.

I completed the necessary forms and signed the Death Certificate and never confused a Coroner's Jury with supercilious details. They were able to come to a logical conclusion without my technicalities.

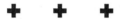

My being on loan from the Royal Canadian Army Medical Corps to the Columbia Coast Mission for one month dragged on for four and a half months. My Colonel had taken his discharge, so no one else knew about me. A "tidy" clerk had placed my records into an inactive file; therefore from the army's point of view I no longer existed.

This information was extended to the paymaster corps; hence no cheques were prepared and I didn't get paid.

Pay from the Columbia Coast Mission was even slower, as they didn't have the funds. Only after I had taken my discharge from the army, was married and we had a child, did I receive my pay from them.

However, eventually we got the army records back to an active status and I was posted back to Military District XI, Vancouver, Little Mountain Military Camp. I hitched a ride back to Vancouver on the police boat, which Sgt. Bill was bringing south for repairs and maintenance. The next day we arrived at the dock in Vancouver and I took a taxi up to my mother's home. It was fortunate she was home as I had insufficient funds for cab fare. My illicit dental practice had not been that lucrative lately.

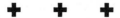

Returning to Vancouver gave me the opportunity to participate in the busy switchboard activities at Infants' Hospital. It was inevitable that

Miss Marriott and I resume our acquaintance. Her clearheaded expressiveness intrigued me.

We started seeing a lot of each other. These visits took place in the evenings, often well into the next morning. This lady had a mind of her own and used it for our long-ranging, in-depth conversations. Things were getting serious, yet neither of us felt our careers included marriage, maybe eventually, but not then. So we broke off our relationship – for one night.

That night I phoned her suite in the hospital to tell her something important about a new bike I was getting. She had said she was going to get caught up with her laundry. She was out. She had gone out with one of the interns!

Later she said she had become restless, he had invited, so she went.

At 6:30 the next morning, I called her. Nursing shifts changed at 7 a.m. and she was a stickler for starting the shift change report at 7 a.m. sharp.

I said, "Enough of this damned nonsense! We're going out tonight when you come off duty. I'll pick you up at six o'clock. Okay?"

Affirmative answer.

We went out that night and every night thereafter. Most of the evenings ended well into early morning. Since these late nights or early mornings were interrupting our sleep, we decided we should get married. We needed some sleep.

This was 1946 and Ruth, although a graduate, had to get permission from the hospital to marry and she also had to find a replacement. The hospital authorities told her she could not continue to work at Infants' as a nurse on the wards since she had been Matron. Such illogical personnel policies persisted even though there was an acute shortage of nurses.

They even tried to cause me problems, suggesting I had gone to Infants' and stolen a nurse to marry, rather that concentrating my efforts on nurses in the main hospital, the Vancouver General.

Really! I may have been one of their interns and one of their residents, and while at one time they owned most of me, they couldn't have my soul!

Without telling Ruth, I had written her parents informing them that I was courting their eldest daughter and telling them of our many trips on my bike. This caused an immediate telephone call to Ruth. Among other things her mother wanted to know, "Do you load and unload on the bike in front of the hospital?" Her mother thought that would be undignified. After that, we tried loading a block from the hospital, but as we drove by, the staff were hanging out the windows waving at us. Thereafter, we loaded in front of the hospital.

My letter to her parents sparked an immediate trip to Vancouver by Mr. and Mrs. Marriott to investigate the matter. Mr. Marriott was frequently there on business, but I'm sure my letter hastened his schedule. This was an important meeting and I wasn't sure what to wear. I finally decided to wear my formal uniform and a Sam Brown belt. For the uninitiated, this is the broad brown waist belt with a narrow belt worn diagonally across one shoulder. It makes a dress uniform more formal. My heart and soul were in this meeting, however I need not have worried. They were wonderful people.

After returning to Calgary, the rest of the family, two brothers and two sisters, wanted to know, "What's he like?" My future mother-in-law was quite effusive; my future father-in-law quite pragmatic: "We'll see how he wears!"

They became my closest friends, I was completely accepted into this marvellous family from day one.

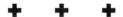

During our courtship we met a charming couple, who lived on a small farm up the Fraser River from New Westminster. Their small daughter had been a patient in Infants' Hospital. The family became friends with Ruth, the hospital matron. They knew we were courting and using a motorcycle as wheels. They issued an open invitation to drop in, if our travels took us in their direction.

Several weeks later we dropped into their gorgeous ranch-style bungalow on a large acreage. Fascinating views of the marine traffic on the Fraser River perpetually played out in front of the living room windows of their home, set on a high point of land. Natural forest shrubs and flowers flowed to the rear of their home. It was a superb location, the house had been admirably planned and set in this idealistic paradise.

They invited us to partake of a "Pot Luck" supper. We were asked to select our own steaks from their walk-in freezer. The scrumptious meal was served on fine bone Spode china, set on a lace tablecloth. If this was "Pot Luck," I mused, what would a formal dinner be.

The husband was a senior official with the MacMillan Bloedel Ltd. organization and, I presumed, involved with basic logging. As we talked in the evening, he was interested in employing me to plan and supervise the first aid and accident prevention operation for their many camps. This elicited superficial interest. Some days later I had exciting speed boat trips to several camps and was able to make worthwhile recommendations. It was a means of repaying their hospitality; as a long term job, my interest was insufficient to justify accepting their offer, and the intrigue would only have been temporary. It was my initial brush with industrial medicine.

✚ ✚ ✚

Ruth and I were married in St. Stephen's Anglican Church, Calgary, by Archdeacon Swanson on August 16, 1946. It was the most fortunate day of my life. "Swanny" had known the Marriott family since Ruth was in her early teens. He had been the clergyman of St. Stephen's, before accepting the call to Christ Church Cathedral in downtown Vancouver. He had known and buried my father in 1945.

When we asked him to perform the service for us, he first insisted on coming out to see the bike; with wartime rationing, he was servicing his parish on a 98 c.c. Francis-Barnett, almost a motorized bicycle. He and I had also met when I worked for the Columbia Coast Mission. Fortunately for us, he was coming to Calgary to marry his daughter, Bea. This was to take place the day after our anticipated date. He said he would be pleased to marry us in his previous church.

After the formal part of our services, we were in the vestry signing the registry when he offered his advice. He probably said this to all new couples, but it impressed me. He was teasing and serious when he told us:

"Now you two, the secret of a successful marriage is for you each to put in 60% – that leaves 20% in excess to overcome friction." It stuck in my mind as a good foundation.

I now had two brothers-in law and two sisters-in-law. My father-in-law, a miller by trade and a salesman by temperament, clicked with me from the start. He was direct and honest – we never had a misunderstanding. My mother-in-law was loving, caring, straightforward and compassionate; thus started a remarkable relationship.

We had an exciting honeymoon, the first evening spent in the Palliser Hotel where I had earlier delivered my luggage. When we entered the room, it dawned on me that Ruth's luggage was locked in the trunk of our new Nash, which I had parked earlier in a garage near the hotel.

I had paid the attendant handsomely to guard our new car. My caution was motivated by knowing that friends had their engine ruined by some prankster pouring syrup into the gas tank. Now I had to return to the garage late at night and generously bribe another attendant to allow me to get Ruth's bags out of our car.

The confusion was relieved when "Room Service" delivered a midnight supper, complete with flowers; I was going to do this right. We had started our life together.

The next morning, as a prank, Ruth called her mother saying, "This is Mrs. Ibberson." The initial reply was, "Oh, yes Pearl, wasn't the wedding and reception delightful," then, "Oh Ruth, you fool!" as they both dissolved in giggles and laughter.

Ruth then phoned my mother and said, "Good morning, this is Mrs. Ibberson." There was dead silence for several seconds until my mother mentally shifted gears and comprehended the meaning of the statement. Then she said, "I have been trying to get you two, but the hotel switchboard wouldn't connect me to your room!" Ruth quickly explained that I had asked the hotel to hold any calls, because I was worried about pranksters.

We honeymooned in Banff and Jasper and returned to Calgary, then went to Saskatoon to see old friends and drove north to Emma Lake where my folks had built a cabin. We then returned to Calgary.

Mr. Marriott would open the front door and say, in jest, "My Gawd, not you two again."

We drove back to Vancouver and, because there was no housing available, we constructed a suite in the basement of my mother's home on Quesnel Drive.

We were able to look back on how we had shared the beauty of the Rocky Mountain Parks and the vastness of the prairies. We had enjoyed housekeeping in many different cabins and shared beautiful sunrises and sunsets.

One morning in a cabin at the foot of Takakaw Falls in the Kicking Horse Pass, we awakened to see our breath – startling in August. I got up and started a fire in the drum stove. Ruth kicked the stove door shut and whoosh, her foot was no longer covered by her nylon stocking; it had melted and vanished.

We had started on that long and fascinating journey of sharing personal experiences. Many things only a couple can understand, some joyful and some sorrowful. The intertwining and interweaving of our lives in marriage. I wish all couples could be as blessed as we have been.

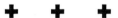

After Army discharge, my post graduate training continued as a staff member of Shaughnessy Veterans Hospital. We were putting together battered bodies and minds. As the troops returned from the Pacific operation, we acquired a large number of patients who had been Japanese prisoners-of-war. What a shocking eye-opener these men were, extremely malnourished physically and mentally. Many weighed less than seventy pounds. They started at the world with a blank unresponsive look. We will never know, in detail, what many went through as they preferred to block most of it out, which is just as well. What is past, is past.

Initially, we thought we just had to feed them. In several days we had a ward of extremely sick men suffering from nausea, vomiting, diarrhea, sweats and nightmares. At someone's suggestion, we asked a senior pediatrician to see these men who were now much sicker than when admitted to hospital. It was a feeding problem so who better to see them than a pediatrician?

Dr. Joe Grant came, examined our patients and then called us together. Joe was an excellent clinician and many of us had been on his service during our training days. We knew he did not suffer fools kindly. His opening remarks got our attention.

"Where in God's name did you guys put your brains?" he said. "These men have been trying to survive on a daily handout of a small bit of rice, if they were lucky. As a result, their gastro-intestinal tracts have reverted to an infant-like state of physiology. You bring them in here and feed them a rich, adult diet. What did you expect their G.I. tracts to do other than revolt and spew it out both ends? That's what a baby would do!" He continued, "That is not the way I trained you fellows. For God's sake, start using the brains He gave you and make these men well!" He was annoyed, with good cause. "Now start thinking and come up with something to help these patients of yours."

That set us back on our heels. We went to work for most of that night and invented a formula for adults, an "infant" adult feeding formula, later adapted by one of the pharmaceutical companies for geriatric use and special sports needs.

The recovery of these patients was miraculous. After a few days on the formula, they were able to handle solids and then made a speedy progression to a well-balanced diet. In no time their lost weight was recovered, exercise re-toned their muscles, their mental outlook improved and they were ready for the next step in rehabilitation.

Our success was due to the wisdom of Dr. Joe Grant, an excellent teacher who made us think. I'm not sure he ever received the credit he deserved, except in our hearts.

About this time I was working on the urological service (prostates, kidney stones, etc.) and my weight was rapidly sneaking up. I was at least ten to fifteen pounds over my usual base line weight. Of course, I was blaming this on Ruth's excellent cooking, not on my excessive intake. In an effort to get control of the situation, she made a recipe of cookies and cut them out with a thimble. As a joke, she sent a package to her father; he wrote back thanking her for the cough drops.

The weight gain had passed the humorous stage when one day she phoned me on the hospital ward. The head nurse, a Miss MacKenzie, in passing the phone over said to Ruth, "As a matter of fact, he is right here, having a patient's special milk shake supplement off the nutrition cart while he is writing up his charts." When I came on the line, Ruth said, "You are having a patient's milk shake! No wonder you are gaining weight. It has nothing to do with my cooking!"

When I investigated, I discovered one milk shake supplement was at least 700 calories; no wonder the pounds were showing on my frame.

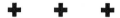

During my time on staff at Shaughnessy hospital our eldest son Bill was born. At birth, a blood incompatibility made him desperately ill, resulting in permanent brain damage, cerebral palsy. We were presented with a large hospital bill. Even though this was the hospital where Ruth trained and in which I had interned, the bottom line was a debt of $1500. My salary was $135 per month. We had an obvious cash shortfall, which begged correction.

Arrangements were made for me to take leave for a month; motivated by desperation, I needed to work several jobs at once.

Fortune smiled on me. Dr. Harry Cannon needed help at Abbotsford. Dr. Shelley Rothwell wanted someone to oversee his practice in the afternoons in New Westminster and a doctor in Haney needed someone to run an evening clinic. These three locations were all within the Fraser Valley.

I kissed my bride good-bye, saying I would see her in a month. My plan was to sleep in whichever doctor's home was the closest at the end of the day. Running three practices in different locations was an exhausting pace, but I was young and needed little sleep. If the young needed sleep, romance would never flourish and it was romance that had resulted in our son's birth and the consequent unanticipated hospital bill. Each physician paid me $500 for covering their practice, a total of $1500.

With pride I paid the Vancouver General Hospital in full. Apart from hospital practice and army medicine, these medical practices were my baptism in the world of "real medicine," I was fortunate to have had the guidance of Dr. Harry Cannon in Abbotsford.

Two episodes pop into my mind. The office was located on the main street, directly above a café. One of the young waitresses came for a consultation. She was complaining of a severe productive cough and an elevated temperature. Examination revealed she had pneumonia. She was put on one of the antibiotics we had at that time, probably an early sulphanilamide and an expectorant cough syrup – she left.

Later that evening when speaking to Ruth on the phone, I mentioned this patient and said an unusual thing had happened in the office. The waitress had forgotten her brassiere. I have not forgotten Ruth's reply,

"Any girl who needs one doesn't forget it." I was naive, but I was learning!

Late one evening a farmer called with an emergency and wanted me to make a country call. "No problem," said I. "Which side of the road are you on, right or left? Hang a lantern on the gate so I can find the place."

Off I went, rushing into the night, always watching the right side of the road for the lantern on a gate. I drove for miles with no sight of a lantern on a gate. Soon I noticed the trucks and cars I was passing had State Washington license plates.

My Gawd. I had driven out of Canada by the back roads and was now in the U.S.A.; the Yanks are hospitable people but they don't appreciate visitors by the back roads. About turn and return to my own country.

Retracing my steps, I found the lantern on the gate. The farmer, facing into town when he called, said right, with me mentally facing out of town when taking his call, his right became my left. I can't remember the emergency, but the lesson of the lantern on the gate saved me hours by thereafter asking for explicit directions when making a country call.

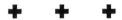

The phrase "Locums Tenens" is the latin phrase meaning temporarily taking someone else's place, literally, standing in their place. The phrase is used by doctors and clergy to specify a temporary replacement. My explanation is needed since latin is no longer a pre-med requisite, although the present generation make frequent use of the term, usually shortened to locums.

Early in one's career, locums pays the rent and sometimes earns amenities. I did many locums on the west coast, transported by that big silver Harley Davidson motorcycle, my little black medical bag carried in one of the leather saddle bags slung across the back fender.

CHAPTER IV
Doctor and Dentist

As work continued at Shaughnessy Hospital, I became more involved in reconstructive surgery. We were repairing badly damaged and often severely burned bodies. I noticed, in doing head and neck repairs, that dental surgeons were not on the hospital staff. They seemed uncomfortable working with patients under general anesthetic in the operating room. To appreciate this today, we must think back forty-five to fifty years. The specialty of plastic surgery was developing as a result of war injuries, like airmen shot down in planes and sailors who jumped in burning fuel oil. Antibiotics and improved anesthetic methods were developing which make this type of surgery possible. The developments and progress within the last fifty years are unbelievable, even for those of us fortunate to have lived through them!

To handle the challenges of Maxillo-Facial surgery it seemed dental training was necessary. This was a completely new field. Since my father had been a dentist and oral surgeon, I had the advantage of background, but I deeply missed being able to seek his counsel in looking at this problem. I wrote to centres teaching this new field and was accepted at Ann Arbor, Michigan, a world class centre. Unfortunately the American authorities did not allow me the privilege of writing my American Medical Board Examinations for an American license, necessary to practice in the U.S.A. This would only be possible if we signified our intentions of becoming American citizens. It was post-war and they were a little protective of American privileges. I did not want to become an American citizen and neither did Ruth. As a consequence, we could not accept this opportunity at Ann Arbor.

I was, however, accepted by the University of Alberta, Edmonton, into their first year dental program on the four year dental degree course. We summoned our courage, packed our few belongings and moved to Edmonton.

The University student body at that time was full of veterans, many married with families. They had singleness of purpose, having spent years away fighting a war, and they were there to complete an education which could support them.

We veterans were older, serious and more mature than the usual students. This came as somewhat of a shock to one of the older professors, a clinician whose teaching was inadequate. We quickly formed a committee of three to present our views and recommendations to the Dean. This committee was made up of senior officer material: an ex-Lt. Commander of the Royal Canadian Navy, an ex-Wing Commander R.C.A.F. and an ex-Major R.C.A.M.C., Army. We paraded before the Dean, came to attention, succinctly presented our views, about turned and marched out. The Dean was speechless, but paid attention to our recommendations and replaced the inadequate teacher. These students were a new breed.

This was long before any Health Insurance schemes and many veterans had young families and minimal income. For this reason, I ran an early morning "Well Baby Clinic" in the basement of the old Med-Dent Building. We examined infants and children, changed formulas, treated colds and coughs and generally separated the unwell from the really sick. The sick were sent over to the University pediatric clinic. No fees were charged, we were all surviving together.

After some searching, Ruth, Bill and I arranged to share the home of a retired widower, Mr. Calhoune, who had worked for Purity Flour Mills. It was a small bungalow with a dugout for a basement. It was located on the south side of Edmonton near the railway tracks and several blocks from Whyte Avenue. The floor plan was old-fashioned, a small parlor in front and a large dining room in the centre, two bedrooms off the dining room, a small kitchen, pantry and bathroom. There was a small bedroom off the kitchen which Mr. Calhoune used. We were about two miles from the University, close enough to walk. This was necessary because we had to sell our new car to pay for dental instruments and tuition.

We paid Mr. C., as we affectionately called him, $50 per month rent and boarded him. Our Department of Veteran Affairs credits were $90 per month. We were not rich, but with Mr. C.'s manifold kindnesses we survived. If he wanted a special cut of meat or special seafood, he quietly provided it.

He was a wonderfully kind man, a millwright by trade. His wife had suddenly died the night before their son, an R.C.A.F. bomber pilot, returned from his first tour of duty. He returned overseas for a second tour of duty and was shot down returning from a bombing raid. Mr. C. received no further information about his only child.

During our two years as Mr. C.'s guests, his health deteriorated and he died toward the end of our second year.

I have never known anyone with more quiet faith than this wonderful man. He knew he was dying and he not only believed, he knew that he would be reunited with his wife and their only child. He would finally learn what had happened to his son.

His kindness extended beyond his death. He had a specific clause in his will allowing us to stay in the house until I finished my University training. It wasn't long because I compressed my third and fourth years into a single year.

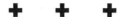

Between my first and second year in dental school, I spent the summer, four-and-a-half months, practicing medicine in Westlock. Westlock is a town about sixty miles northeast of Edmonton. I worked for Dr. George Whissell.

When we moved to Westlock, we took over Dr. Frank Woodman's home. This home had a unique water system, a well, piped into the house. For us city types, this was quite different. Before he left for post-graduate training, Frank lowered a burning blow torch into the well to thaw the frozen intake pipe. There had been a minor explosion, since the well was filled with gasoline fumes. Frank lost his eyebrows and moustache and the blow torch full of gasoline fell to the bottom of the well. For days I burped gasoline-tasting material. I was afraid to light a cigarette. Then the well went dry.

In the country, you can't phone the city services department, so you develop your own solution. Three hundred gallons of fresh water dumped into the well disappeared. Where it went, we never knew. We repeated this three times. Three times it disappeared. Each tank cost $10. This was costly and not the solution to the problem. To provide for our drinking and cooking needs, I was transporting two one-gallon jugs to and from the hospital each day. For other water needs, such as plumbing, we set up a horse trough outside and ran the intake pipe into this container. It was soon covered with green algae and other residents. The system worked well, within limits. Each time one of us was using the "facilities," the call went out: "Does anyone want to get in on this flush?"

Frank was not the handyman type, in fact, quite the contrary. I sometimes wondered just how he had mastered the art of using a razor each morning. Everything in that house needed fixing.

Ruth correctly smelled mice in the kitchen. They came in through the broken door which was used to pass wood for the kitchen stove. The house had been wired long after initial construction and the electrical outlets were flush with the floor. When the creek overflowed and flooded the house, the electrical outlets filled with silt. Frank couldn't understand why they didn't work. Off with the power, lots of vacuuming and picking and then they worked.

The aluminum kitchen counter edge strip was held at one end by a single screw. In order to open a drawer or get into a lower cupboard, one had to hold up the whole strip. For want of several screws, the kitchen had driven his wife crazy.

My wife would not put up with it. The repair was made the first morning before I went to the hospital!

At the end of the first week in our new home, I went rushing upstairs and the whole handrail came off in my hand. It almost went through the window on the landing. It was so ridiculous, we both collapsed with laughter. After this episode, we started at the top and went through each floor of the house until we reached the basement. We carried out dozens of minor repairs to make the house habitable. Ruth wasn't surprised by this. Frank had grown up in Calgary, in the house behind hers. He was a friend of her brothers and he just wasn't Mr. Fixit.

The house had a brand new coal and wood stove in the kitchen. Ruth and I were not used to such a stove, having both been brought up in the city. Some days the stove worked beautifully, other days nothing went right. Through sheer stubbornness, Ruth once took three days to cook scalloped potatoes. They were not edible, but they were finally cooked.

Several days later, my mother-in-law (whom I always referred to as my "interfering mother-in-law" because she never did) came for a visit. She had grown up in rural Manitoba. When I told her of our temperamental stove and how I had cleaned the pipes and flue, she said, "Don't be ridiculous, I grew up with one of these stoves." She went outside and said, "If you cut down that big branch growing into the chimney, it should work fine." She was right.

It also explained why the stove was temperamental. One end of the clothesline was attached to that tree and the fence at the other end of the yard. The weight of the clothes pulled the branch out of the chimney. Laundry days were days when the stove worked. When the wind blew in a certain direction, the chimney was temporarily clear, and the stove worked. After removing the branch, our stove worked perfectly. "City types" have a lot to learn in the country.

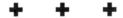

One morning after rounds at the hospital, Dr. Whissell said, "I want you to make a call out to Mr. Simms' farm. I will tell you exactly how to get there."

He always gave explicit directions and did not believe in wasting time by getting lost. He knew the countryside in detail. "Don't get temperamental on me," he clearly said. "You are going out there to sew up an injured bull. Keep in mind that bull is more important to that farmer than one of his children. The bull cost $10 000. He reckoned he could always get another child, but he couldn't afford another bull!"

These farmers were forgiving people, steady and patient. They never let on they were aware of my carrying several textbooks in the glove compartment. When I made an excuse to get another instrument from my second bag, they didn't look as I frantically thumbed through the pages to refresh my memory or to look up the dose of a seldom used drug. Bless them! These are the kind of people I think of when the church celebrates All Saints Day.

After driving twenty miles, following directions, I arrived at the farm and met the largest bull I have ever seen. He was big, very big. He reminded me of a tank. During the war, I had some experience with tanks. My experience with bulls, however, was minimal. This monster had torn his chest open by rushing into a barbed-wire fence, motivated by desire. Isn't it amazing the amount of trouble racing hormones cause in the world?

The farmer's sons assured me they could immobilize this monster by using stanchions. I hoped they were right, since I would be immediately in front of him.

The boys seemed to have no difficulty immobilizing the bull and told me it was safe to examine the wound. It was nasty, but clean and should come together without too much trouble. Boy, that animal was big, and all male. My apprehension caused me to put more than enough local anesthetic into the wound. It was important that the animal feel no pain, particularly since I was to be in his line of sight. After putting in at least sixty stitches, the job was finished. I heaved a sigh of relief that I had not been trampled.

"Well Doc," the farmer said, "that looks like a neat professional job. How much?"

"I have no idea of the charge," I replied. "We'll leave that up to Dr. Whissell. I'm working on salary this summer, taking Dr. Frank Woodman's place, while he is away on a post-graduate course."

It must have been the correct response. His next comment was, "Put your bag in the car, come up to the house where you can clean up and the wife will find you some coffee and pie. Thank's for fixing my prize bull."

My hat goes off to the veterinarians who handle similar problems all the time. I'm not easily intimidated, but a living, breathing, snorting tank with horns! Really!!

If you wonder why I was doing this job, it was because veterinarian surgeons were not readily available in the country in those days.

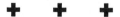

As weeks passed, I became busy with obstetrics. It was frustrating, annoying and scary when these ladies, having received no pre-natal care, presented themselves in labor to be admitted to the hospital. I had no knowledge of their past history, no previous examination to guide me, I knew nothing about them. Fortunately, most of them were healthy, young farm women who considered childbirth a normal, natural thing, which it is when there are no complications. My imagination feared the worst.

I was mumbling about this state of affairs when Ruth, who is smarter than me and always goes for the solution, said, "If this upsets you so much, why don't you do something about it? Why don't you start a pre-natal clinic at the hospital, Sundays after church? Most of these girls come in to attend Mass."

We set up a pre-natal clinic in the hospital after Mass. I became aware of potential obstetrical problems and acquired the best collection of pies, cakes, pickles and other assorted goodies. This seemed to solve most of the problems, but not all.

One young farm wife arrived in labor and produced an infant in record time. Resuscitation of the infant presented some problems, it was hard to get the infant to breathe. In addition, in the middle of this emergency the mother had a severe post partum hemorrhage. She was bleeding like a ruptured fire hose. I was extremely busy with these emergencies, which I'm happy to report we eventually controlled.

As I stepped out of the delivery room into the small waiting area and met her twenty year-old husband, I said,

"We had a bit of a bad time in there. Your wife is fine now, but she had a severe hemorrhage. Oh, and the baby is now breathing well."

"Gee, thanks Doc. I was kinda worried. It took longer than the last time. You sure she's going to be okay?"

"Yes, quite sure," I replied.

"Oh, by the way, Doc, what did we have? Not twins I hope."

I was thunderstruck. I had no idea whether the child was male or female. I had been so busy getting that baby delivered quickly. The infant needed oxygen before brain damage occurred; and then with that terrifying bleed, I doubt I had even looked. I couldn't recall. With two lives at risk, it didn't seem that important to me. It was important to the father, however. I felt totally inadequate.

I started to answer him. "It was a...maybe...it was...a..." The Catholic sister from the case room pulled the back of my gown and whispered, "It was a boy."

"Oh yes," I said, "Sister tells me it was a boy. A healthy, big boy."

The father, with an incredulous look, said, "Geez, Doc, can't you tell the difference?"

For several weeks thereafter, I was known as "the doctor who can't tell the difference." As I would walk out of the clinic at noon or in the evening, there were always a few "hands" lounging in front to greet me with: "Hey, Doc, come out to the farm, we got some heifers and steers so we can teach you the difference."

It only took about six weeks to settle down. Then they were on to someone or something else. If you're going to be stupid you develop a thick skin.

As the practice expanded, we continued with babies and went on to remove chronic large infected tonsils and adenoids. For a time, I was the Tonsillectomy King. We would book these kids in batches in the operating room for their T's and A's (tonsillectomies and adenoidectomies).

The families would come into town early in the morning. We would do the surgery. The other members of the family would have a picnic on the front lawn of the hospital. We would check these kids after finishing at the office. If they were fine with no sign of bleeding, we discharged them. We requested a return office visit in one week as a follow-up. I don't recall any of them having a post-operative bleed.

My biggest problem was proving to the parents that these children could eat afterwards. They would appear in the office one week after surgery wrapped in a scarf in the middle of summer. Their pink faces were bathed in perspiration, their tongues hanging out like a panting dog. There had to be a way to convince their parents they could eat and there was! There was only one drug store in town and they had a soda fountain. I hit upon the idea of writing a specific prescription for these kids. I had a special name for my prescription, "Ban. Sp't #278. Use no substitutions." The parents would take the prescription to the pharmacist in good faith. He would rush around in the soda fountain and produce a banana split. The child ate. I was a hero. The parents were convinced. They all went home and life continued.

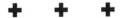

To the north of Westlock, on a gravel road, was the hamlet of Flatbush. Since there was no drug store, when I went there each Wednesday afternoon, I took boxes of pharmaceutical samples in my car. En route, I would stop when I passed the local road grader. He was an ulcer patient. Our consultation and examinations were carried out roadside. His treatment varied with what samples were available in my travelling pharmacy, but we eventually healed his ulcer.

The working facilities in Flatbush included a single shack of unfinished two-by-fours which supported the siding, a heating system consisting of a single pot-bellied stove and water facilities of a pail, basin and slop pail. These facilities were primitive, but effective.

I would examine and treat patients all afternoon. Some were simple cases, some complex. While I was there, I did the labwork. The more complex cases were brought into the clinic in Westlock. Abscesses, we opened and drained. Teeth beyond repair, we extracted. Fractures were set and casted. Lacerations were repaired.

I recall one young lad coming in with a severe laceration of his foot. He had stepped on a broken bottle in the creek. I explained that by injecting local anesthetic we could repair and suture his wound without pain. While inserting the stitches, he vocalized a blow-by-blow description to his mother and all other patients waiting to see me. That's advertising!

My employer, Dr. Whissell, believed in making medical services available to patients he knew would be hesitant. Unless it was an emergency, most of them would not take time from their jobs or farms to see a doctor. He correctly realized that taking medical care to patients eliminated some possible future emergencies by practicing prevention and early treatment. If the situation required more treatment than we could provide, we hospitalized the patient in Westlock.

Westlock was a wonderful introduction to the realistic practice of medicine without hand-holding and without specialists willing to assume every responsibility. Patient problems were real; you had to make the diagnosis and do something in the way of treatment. You saw these people every day in town and the responsibility for their medical needs was on your shoulders.

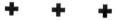

The Sisters of Charity at the Immaculata Hospital in Westlock were a wonderful, caring group of women who supported us through a time of sorrow. Our second child, a boy, was born prematurely in Edmonton. Ruth had been making the trip to Edmonton weekly for Rh antibody checks at the Red Cross blood lab and pre-natal checks with her obstetrician. When Bill, our first boy, was born, we encountered a rare Rh incompatibility problem which caused a breakdown of blood cells and resultant brain and nerve damage, causing him to have severe cerebral palsy. Ruth's antibody levels had been climbing, but we were hopeful that awareness of the problem and early treatment would give us a normal child.

Labor pains started late one evening, some weeks before the estimated due date. Dr. Whissell was away and I was the only doctor available for the clinic. Ruth was sent to Edmonton by ambulance. Unfortunately, I could not accompany her, making us both apprehensive.

Bill and I were up early the next morning since I was booked for a full morning of surgery. After he had been bathed and fed, we got to the hospital at 7:15 a.m. The first Sister we met heard our story. She clutched Bill to her loving bosom and the two of them disappeared into the nun's living quarters. I did not see him for about eight days, but knew he was well cared for. Meanwhile, they fed me dinner each night.

Ruth's labor continued and she was given a low spinal anesthetic for the delivery of a second son. Initially everything looked stable, although Ruth expressed concerns about this child. Her concerns were real and our son died on the fifth day.

She had to go through this heartbreaking trial alone. I was trapped in Westlock as the only doctor available for the clinic. There were phone calls, but I felt inadequate not being with her in this time of sorrow. I could not have made a difference to the outcome, but I have always felt she needed my hand to grip and my shoulder to cry on, neither of which were there.

Sometimes, one of the complications of a spinal anesthetic is a post-spinal headache. Ruth's headache persisted for 21 days. After a week in the University Hospital where the maternity ward was an old army barracks, we felt she would be more comfortable and things might return to normal more rapidly if we transferred her to the Immaculata Hospital in Westlock. The Sisters insisted on a private room. She had been in a four-bed maternity ward at the University Hospital.

The Sisters not only insisted on looking after our son, but also my wife and me. Every evening when I had finished at the office, they served us supper in Ruth's room. They were considerate, thoughtful and good to us. They would not accept payment other than our insurance. Nothing for a private room or extra care, nor babysitting and husband-feeding.

Theirs was a very strict order. They were not allowed to eat in our presence and they could not accept an invitation to receive hospitality in our home, unless someone was mortally ill. Ruth said she was willing to climb back into bed in feigned illness, but mortal illness was too much.

We were allowed to drive two of the Sisters to a nearby town and buy them an ice cream cone. On the way back, they saw wild raspberry bushes and insisted on picking berries for the patients. When we got them back to the hospital, we were asked to stay for supper, even though they could not eat with us. One could never repay their kindness.

Eventually we were allowed to buy a small autoclave (sterilizer) for the hospital's operating room.

They truly lived their goodness and kindness.

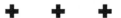

As Fall and the Labor Day weekend approached, an interesting drama unfolded. A new urban-trained bank manager had come to town and introduced hard, inflexible rules to collect money owed to the bank. Over the long weekend someone, no one knew exactly who (there were rumors), had backed several large grain trucks up to the bank, poked a hole in one of the high windows, inserted a grain auger and filled the bank to a depth of four feet. There was grain everywhere, even in the drawers. On top of this pile of grain was a large note:

"I DON'T HAVE ANY MONEY. THIS IS ALL I'VE GOT. YOU SHOVEL IT OUT. YOU TRY TO SELL IT."

No one ever took credit nor blame for this episode. The town's folk were on the side of the perpetrator. Farmers are long-suffering, but there are limits. The bank manager was transferred the next day.

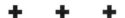

University dental school resumed in September, 1948. I was registered to complete the remaining classes and labs in third year and simultaneously complete my fourth and final year. This would allow for graduation with a doctorate degree in dental surgery (D.D.S.) in May, 1949.

We returned to Mr. Calhoune's cottage and resumed our busy academic life. It is not difficult to take two years of university courses in one term. All it takes is excellent organization and the help of your fellow students to take carbon paper notes in the classes you can't attend because of a conflict in timing. You cannot afford the luxury of feeling sorry for yourself. We looked forward to returning to dental school. Most of the labs and technical matters were behind us and now the clinical aspect of dealing with patients was paramount. This was the exciting part. This was to be the end point of all the planning and economic sacrifice.

Classes and clinics went well and my Christmas exam marks were in the top ten of the class. I detected a sense of confusion on the part of the senior dental clinicians and the Dean, however, in how to handle me. I was aiming at acquiring a degree and willing to fulfil the requirements, but we all knew I did not intend to practice general dentistry, i.e. filling cavities, doing bridgework and making dentures.

I was an enigma. The Dean was doing major dental and maxillo-facial surgery in the University Hospital, but felt he should use the hospital interns as assistants. As I had put in several more years as a surgical intern and resident than other interns, I wondered why he didn't use me as a surgical assistant. I wanted more training in the field of oral surgery. The interns were only interested in general surgery. I soon learned the dental school had never finalized the planning of my training. Maybe I should have gone about the matter through the medical school?

The truth of the matter is, this was a time of educational reorganization for everyone. Post-war educational demands were vast. Specialties were being born. I was probably premature in asking for training in maxillo-facial surgery, a specialty which was not yet clearly defined.

Meanwhile we faced an economic problem. We did not have enough funds to see us through to graduation. We had sold and eaten our new car and other saleable assets, converting them into books, dental instruments and tuition.

I had gone to one of the banking institutions on Edmonton's south side and explained my situation and tried to arrange a loan of two-hundred dollars. I had plenty of education, great potential, would probably be a top earner, had a past history of financial responsibility, but no line of credit and no collateral. Citing excellent references made no difference.

Without collateral, no loan.

It proved my first belief about the banking business; if you can prove that you don't need the money and have collateral to cover their risk, they are anxious to do business with you. If you are desperate for a loan and have no collateral, they can't do business. The alternative is to see 'Loan Sharks', for me not an alternative.

In the past, when single, I had been broke and it was a minor problem, rectified by taking on another job. Being broke when married with a family to support and being too busy to handle another job, was something quite serious. We were not completely broke. We had our last $19 and no cash flow.

Our problem list was increased by the beginnings of a third pregnancy for Ruth. Unfortunately her antibody titre was rising at an alarming rate. We were worried and consultations resulted in a decision to terminate the pregnancy and finalize the Rh problems with a sterilizing tubal ligation. Since this was before the days of any available Health Care Insurance, being broke, we felt insecure and vulnerable.

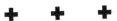

I do believe "The Man Upstairs" hears our prayers, particularly those of desperation. Out of the blue I received a phone call from the assistant medical director of Imperial Oil Limited in Toronto, saying they required a physician to go to Norman Wells, N.W.T., to be responsible for their employees and operate the hospital at the refinery site. They would supply transportation, food, utilities and a small house, plus salary of $500 per month. I was speechless! They seemed to know of my training. They were employing me as a physician, however, if I wished to practice dentistry in my off hours that was my business. I would be free to charge patients for my dental services. We were to have no overhead. This was mana from heaven.

There was one embarrassing factor as I accepted this challenge. We were so broke, I had to request a salary advance so I could purchase parkas for Ruth, Bill and me. We couldn't go that far north without adequate clothing. I hadn't even worked for them, yet they advanced the money.

Maybe that is why they are in the petroleum industry, not banking or government.

To make this move we again disrupted the Marriott household. We no longer possessed a car, having eaten it. Ruth's father drove up from Calgary and we loaded the car with our few possessions. Since the three of us were returning to Calgary as a base, we discovered there was no room for dad. This wonderfully supportive father returned on the train. His only comment was a chuckle. We drove to Calgary in the comfort of his automobile. The least we could do was to pick him up at the train station. Without the support of my in-laws, we would not have survived the early years.

Unfortunately, due to lack of funds, we left dental school four months short of meeting graduation requirements.

CHAPTER V
Of Ice and Men

We flew into Norman Wells, North West Territories, which is just south of the Arctic Circle on the MacKenzie River, arriving early in February, 1949 in the company plane, a Lockheed Lodestar, CF-TDB. The temperature was minus sixty-five degrees fahrenheit, with a sixty m.p.h. north wind.

As we were deplaning, with Bill well wrapped up, Ruth gave me a shocked look which spoke volumes, "I have followed you to some pretty crazy places, but this has got to be the worst."

We received a most hospitable welcome as we came off the company aircraft. We were taken to our house and later learned that only the camp superintendent and the camp doctor were assigned a house. Married employees lived in two-room apartments and single employees lived in barrack-like accommodation.

Our house was small, a two-bedroom bungalow with a living room, dining room, bathroom, kitchen with pantry in the back entrance, which served as the main entrance. For some unknown reason, the living room ceiling was sagging and we had to hold it up in order to walk across the room. All of the buildings were set on piles (sections of drill stem pipe). The permafrost prevented digging basements or setting buildings on cement footings, and thawing the ground only made it unstable.

Norman Wells was the site of many natural gas and crude oil wells. During the war, the crude oil was pumped down the Canol pipeline to the refinery in Whitehorse. Shortly after the war, the refinery at Whitehorse was dismantled, trucked to Edmonton and reassembled. When we were at Norman Wells, Imperial Oil's on site refinery manufactured most of the petroleum products sold in the Western Arctic.

Our first night was memorable. Someone had found a large crib for twenty-two month old Bill. It was late, it had been a long day and we were ready for bed. To our horror, all the windows in the house were open at least two or three inches. Given the outside temperature, plus the wind chill factor, we were certain we were going to freeze to death. We slammed all the windows shut, settled Bill in the crib and piled everything we could think of on top of him so he wouldn't freeze. I know he was covered with so much stuff he couldn't turn over. Shortly thereafter, we went to bed. At 2 a.m. we awoke, roasting to death and throwing off all our covers. Poor Bill was bathed in sweat and panting like a dog. We got rid of the extra blankets and covers. We found a butcher knife in the kitchen and spend an hour chipping the ice off the windows and prying them open two or three inches. They were never shut again once we learned about the unique heating system.

The buildings were on piles. Steam generated in the power plant ran in pipes just above the ground and these were covered by a protective roof. Water lines went with the steam pipes so the water didn't freeze. Each building had a wooden skirt from the base of the building to the ground and steam was discharged in a controlled fashion under each building. In essence, we had a radiant heating system through the floors, which gave us the most comfortably heated house we have ever had. Since all the water pipes had to run beside a steam pipe though, we had difficulty getting cold water from the tap. The problem was solved by keeping a large jug of water in the fridge.

We had a comfortable house, the best thus far in our marriage. We had no expenses, the house, the food, the utilities and transportation were supplied. Lots of work and no place to spend money if you didn't drink. What a great opportunity to build a nest egg for the future and that was our plan.

Everyone ate in a common mess hall, which made sense since everyone in the camp worked, with the exception of the superintendent's wife and Ruth. Imperial Oil wouldn't allow Ruth to work for me in the hospital and we were the only couple with a baby.

Since we had a kitchen and a refrigerator at home and an infant, it was often easier to draw cooked or raw food from the mess kitchen. Sunday dinner was one of the occasions that we preferred to eat at home.

We worked six days per week, Sunday being the only day off. The drinking amongst some on Saturday night was phenomenal. If one appeared for work on Monday morning drunk, employment was terminated. Sunday was often a case of the semi-sober trying to assist the completely drunk in order to recover in time for work Monday morning. Parading up and down outside the mess hall, most workers were often half frozen being sick. It was not a situation in which to take an infant when you had a choice.

Our transportation was a three-quarter ton U.S. Army ambulance from the Canol pipeline days. It was the same as the ambulance seen on the TV series M.A.S.H. It had four-wheel drive and springs so firm they never flexed. Fuel came from a 400-gallon tank on legs with a filler hose. No meter and no record of what you used, because there was only one road to the landing strip (two miles) and we manufactured the gasoline. In the cold of winter, if you took a vehicle out of the heated garage, you never shut off the motor. It was safer and easier to keep it running. If you turned it off in that cold weather the oil congealed and the starter couldn't turn the motor over.

+ + +

The day after we arrived, the temperature was still in the minus-sixties. I received a radio message that the R.C.A.F. was picking me up early in the morning to see an injured airman. We were to pick him up at Tuktayuktuk, many miles further north on the edge of the Arctic Ocean. The aircraft was a DC-3 converted for carrying freight. It was cold in that freight car-like fuselage, so I made my way onto the flight deck. The pilot, co-pilot and navigator were not gracious about the presence until I warmed up and started peeling off clothing. I had found the jacket of my old army battle-dress a comfortable, practical piece of clothing under a parka since it had lots of pockets. It still had my medical corps insignia, service ribbons and rank from active service during the war. Once it was apparent that as a major I outranked, by far, all the members of the flight crew, things became very hospitable and I was invited to stay on the flight deck where it was warm. I later learned the reason for the initial cool reception. The plane was carrying some classified radar navigational equipment on board and the crew was uncertain of my security clearance.

At that time of year, with no real sunlight and long black winter nights, we had about twenty minutes of dusk in which to land on the frozen strip at Tuktayuktuk, pick up our patient and become airborne again.

The airman had received some nasty injuries in a sledding accident. After getting his stretcher secured and attending to his injuries with splints, controlling his pain and stabilizing his condition, I again went forward to the flight deck. We had then been airborne about an hour when I said to the crew, "Well fellows, he is well settled down, break out the sandwiches and coffee, I'm starved."

They replied, "Geez, Doc, didn't you get something to eat at the strip when we landed?"

I replied, "You guys know I was too busy checking out the patient and getting him loaded so you could take off in what light there was! Now, let's quit fooling around, I'm hungry!"

The navigator said, "We weren't fooling. The only thing on board is this frozen sandwich left over from a previous flight. I can put it on the radio and thaw it."

As the sandwich thawed, the bread curled up like a steel spring. The baloney just lay there, hard cold and dead. It wasn't much. It wasn't even good, but it was all there was. Even the patient had eaten before we left.

We got back to Norman Wells at midnight which was long after the mess had closed. As I made my way home to our little house, my hunger intensified. Surely we had some food at home. Rummaging around, the only thing I found was a gross of powdered eggs. I knew about powdered eggs from my days in the army. I was hungry, but not that hungry. I went to bed with my empty stomach growling. Morning came and with it a hearty breakfast at the mess hall.

The reason Ruth had been unable to stock the house with basic food items was Bill. While I was flying further north, Bill had become extremely ill, spiking a very high temperature from a severe throat infection. When I first looked at him late in the evening my first thought was diphtheria, even though he had been immunized. Ruth had been busy all day nursing Bill and unable to go to the mess hall for her meals or supplies. Fortunately he responded to antibiotics and fluids, although he had us worried for twenty-four hours.

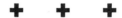

During the first few days, our house developed a maintenance problem. The wall board of the ceiling was coming loose and falling down. Not just the one board we initially encountered; now the entire ceiling was involved. We couldn't continue living there and since the camp was not up to full operational capacity and we were not yet medically busy, we moved into one ward of the hospital, taking Bill's crib with us.

Late one evening, really it was very early morning, 3 a.m. and of course pitch black, Ruth heard some noises and climbed over me in the double bed next to the wall to investigate. Two very drunk natives had stumbled into the hospital looking for a warm dry bed. By the time I awakened and caught up to Ruth, she was reading these natives the Riot Act standing in the centre of the ward in her nightie. They were being dismissed, sent back out into the cold. I pointed out that one of them had no socks, he had removed them as he got into bed. It was minus 60 degrees outside. She didn't care. How dare they crawl into bed in the hospital in their intoxicated state. Out!

Thereafter, as long as we were in the north, whenever Jonas, one of the participants, saw Ruth coming he crossed the street!

During Christmas break, production decreased and most of the staff went "outside" for holidays. The work week was six days and vacation time and a percentage of wages were held back so employees had money to support themselves while on holidays.

Later in my career, I met individuals who had stayed in the Arctic for some years without a break. They were completely self-centred, disinterested in what was transpiring on the outside. The company's rule of "out for holidays" made complete sense.

We were soon building camp up to full strength and full production. As I later learned, everyone had at least three or four jobs. The carpenter was also the barber and the fireman, and so on. When at full strength, the

Imperial Oil camp supported about 250 employees. The only other permanent workers at that time were a small detachment of army signal corps who also functioned as a weather station and a radio message relay unit. As a sideline, they had limited facilities for re-broadcasting music from California. In the winter, we had excellent reception from many parts of the world. Routinely we heard our news from Australia. In the summer, we would only get the small signal corps local station. We had taken up a large library of 78 r.p.m. records to satisfy our musical appetites.

The hospital had been closed during the eight-week December/January period when the refinery was shut down and only a skeleton staff remained in camp. Now it was time to get all equipment and staff operational. Strange how things disappear or get reassigned when no one is around. The initial two weeks of start-up time was spent finding things that had disappeared. A mythical someone moved them. The hospital was no different.

When I took it over, it was a mess. I don't know why. I'm sure that the previous doctor had left it in excellent shape. In those days, everyone had a tendency to help themselves on the basis that we were all inter-dependent. It wasn't stealing, just borrowing, and it probably hasn't changed over the years.

Since this had initially been an American base, in the days of the Canol pipeline, we had prodigious amounts of equipment, much of which did not show itself until spring thaw. We had fields of trucks, parts, desks, filing cabinets, bath tubs, telephones, etc. We even had a large quantity of horse collars. There were no working horses in the western arctic. Some salesman was smooth in his handling of the Americans who were defending our arctic during the war.

In the hospital, I had large quantities of everything, bottles of 1000 tablets of drugs such as sulphathiazole and aspirin and other basic pharmaceuticals, enough equipment to stock a 200 bed institution.

The hospital was a single-storey structure set on the edge of a bay on the MacKenzie River. When fully operational, it consisted of twenty-four beds, a lab, an operating room, a doctor's office and later a dental office and an x-ray and dark room for developing films.

My head nurse, Miss Shirley Babin, had arrived about the same time we had. Shirley was a top-notch head nurse. Her background included training in the operating room, which complemented my surgical skills. Earlier in her career, she had contracted tuberculosis and during her recovery had taken training as an x-ray technician. Our personalities meshed and a great team was born.

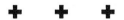

The hospital had grown from a first aid station, but diagnostic x-ray facilities were not part of the picture. The time had come and enquiries were made and bids were submitted for this type of equipment. The successful bid came from a young engineer with Picker X-Ray, Cec Bridgeman. He took the trouble to learn the size of the freight doors and weight capabilities of the company aircraft. His quote was the only one that specified the packaging would fit in the freight bays and the weight of each package. He also arranged to personally travel with these pieces of equipment and carry out installation and calibration of the machine to ensure its proper operation. Thus we acquired a Picker portable 300 MA (milliampere) diagnostic unit and we began a life-long friendship with Cec Bridgeman and his family.

Weather being the deciding factor, we were not sure how long the company aircraft and Cec would be at Norman Wells. We worked all night unpacking, assembling, calibrating and generally installing our one and only diagnostic x-ray unit. For its time, it was an impressive unit. In retrospect, however, it was pretty basic. It worked perfectly on the first attempt. It may have been a fluke, but we preferred to think of it as accurate scientific assembly.

The weather stayed warm and Cec was in the mood for a few days holiday. We had some wonderful picnics as we explored by four wheel drive ambulance and boat our part of the great MacKenzie River.

The production of diagnostic x-ray films requires a source of x-rays to expose film in a cassette holder and then development similar to that of photographic film. A problem in the Arctic, mentioned previously, was getting cold water since the steam lines travel with the water lines. Our cold water was always warm. The temperature of the developer, wash water and fixing solution is critical. If it is too hot, the emulsion with the picture slides off the base of the x-ray film. Fortunately, the quality of films have since improved. Somehow we needed to cool the chemical solutions, but ice cubes, if we had enough, only diluted the solutions.

No problem was too great for the engineering staff at the refinery. They ran a steam tracer line to a small creek three hundred yards away. This prevented the intake pipe from freezing and they built a separate pumping station to continuously circulate water around the coils which wrapped the three chemical tanks. A valve was installed to regulate the rate of water flow. This system allowed the adjustment we needed to control the temperature. I'm not sure what it cost in man hours and equipment, but it worked precisely and we never changed it. We now had diagnostic x-ray facilities. We were on our way to developing an excellent hospital.

Since the steam tracer pipe prevented the creek from freezing, we soon learned the bears considered it thoughtful of us to create their own personal drinking fountain, open year round regardless of temperature. They entertained us with their antics.

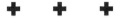

Another problem that worried me was backup lighting. This was particularly inadequate in the operating room and on the wards. How could I fumble around in the dark in the O.R. or with sick patients on the ward using only a flashlight?

The Americans involved in building the Canol pipeline had more equipment stored at Norman Wells than one could imagine. The cost of shipping it south at one dollar per pound, one way, was too expensive, so it was left at Norman Wells. If something was needed, it was probably there.

Fortunately, I found a steam-operated turbine generator, exactly what we needed since we had lots of steam. We hooked up the turbine, did some auxiliary wiring to the operating room, the wards and the halls. When emergency lighting was required, we turned on a large steam valve, closed a knife switch and the auxiliary lighting system glowed, eventually into intense light. We had our back up system. The whine of the turbine resembled a jet engine. It had all the elements of overkill, but it worked.

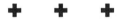

When we moved into our company house, there was a minimum of furniture. The essentials were there, a bed, a crib, a chest of drawers and I recall a kitchen table and some basic kitchen chairs. However, the living room was bare. Rummaging around, which everyone did when in need, I discovered some California redwood in the carpentry shop. With a little ingenuity, I built a coffee table, a sofa and end tables. With a bit more scrounging for odds and ends, our living room was furnished.

The carpentry and machine shops were marvellous places in which to develop what one needed. Once the fellows knew you had skills and would exercise caution while working the machines, you were free to make your own projects in the off hours. We lacked nothing. Skill and ingenuity created what we needed. A few months after arriving in the Arctic, we were living in a very comfortable home.

With the days lengthening, the lack of drapes presented a problem, as we were awakened earlier each day. Ruth wrote Dr. Birrell about this problem and he authorized her to fix it at company expense. Letters passed between Ruth and her Mum who acted as our purchasing agent for drapery material and lining in Calgary. I can't remember where Ruth found a sewing machine in camp, but gorgeous lined drapes were sewn and the house looked magnificent and we didn't waken at four a.m.

As the weeks passed, we settled into a good working routine – up early, breakfast, off to the hospital by 8 a.m. Then see hospital patients, run an office, attend to the lab and x-ray work, do correspondence, carry out public health inspections and in the evening, practice dentistry.

The camp at Norman Wells was very comfortable. Sports and entertainment equipment were complete, including sheets of curling ice and a recreation hall which contained a complete darkroom for amateur photographers. There was no television, as it had not been invented, yet we were spoiled.

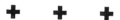

To keep up to date with my profession, I enrolled in a correspondence course in general surgery from McGill University. It was an in-depth reading, question and answer course, preparatory to taking the fellowship examinations from the Canadian Royal College of Surgeons. We had some difficulty smoothing out the correspondence and reply questions. The mail came irregularly, maybe every two or three weeks, sometimes by company plane and sometimes by commercial airlines. Expressions in the north at that time were: "C.P.A. – Can't Promise Anything" and "T.C.A. (referring to TransCanada Airlines, a precursor to Air Canada) – 'Tain't Coming Anyhow." The mail would often get dumped in a snow bank, to accommodate a paying passenger, the thought being that mail could always be taken on the next trip.

My letters to Dr. Birrell, the medical director in Toronto, were numbered to maintain continuity. Mail would come in batches and replies had to be ready in a matter of hours or, if we were lucky and the crew stayed overnight, the next morning. Telephone wires to the outside didn't exist; therefore our correspondence life was a series of mini-crises.

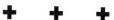

In addition to being the doctor, I had several other jobs. This was normal for frontier medicine. I was also the coroner, the public health officer, the issuer of marriage licenses, the issuer of fur export licenses and Justice of the Peace with the power of two J.O.P.s, I never did understand the significance of the latter, it just said so on the official parchment.

While in Ottawa acquiring these additional powers, a senior civil servant approached me with a confidential departmental problem he thought I might fix. This was in the early days of paying the baby bonus. It had come to his attention that many of the Indians and Eskimos in the western arctic were technically unmarried and they were not exactly sure of the number of their progeny. While I was up there, could I run around as a Justice of the Peace and tidy up the situation by marrying them and counting their children? He had no concept, nor understanding, of the vastness of the Arctic nor the native civilization and customs. I tried to explain that these people were married in their own manner, having undergone a blanket ceremony which was the equivalent of our marriage custom.

Counting the children would be less accurate; as is the custom in many primitive cultures, they sometimes gave their children away and kept track of this in their Oral History. Often the first child was given to the grandparents. The young couple couldn't really cope with a child in their early marriage and the grandparents would need the insurance of young muscles and hunting skills as they aged. The young couple saw nothing wrong in this and when viewed from their point of view and lifestyle, it made sense. Not to this civil servant – it upset his bookkeeping. He wasn't interested in their history or customs, only his bookkeeping.

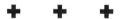

As Public Health Officer, I was called upon one Friday morning to fly with Gordie Latham, senior company pilot, across the nearby mountains. We were to land on a lake where the Indians were gill netting whitefish and piling them like cord wood for our inspection.

I remember saying to Gordie, "Why am I on this flight?"

He said, "As Public Health Officer, you have to certify these fish as fresh before we buy them and take them to camp."

We had taken forty-five gallon drums of gasoline to barter for the fish. It was minus forty-five degrees below zero, with a wind. As the Indians pulled these beautiful whitefish out of the gill nets, they actually froze while they were working with them. They worked in a permanent deep-freeze – the fish could not have been any fresher.

We unloaded the drums of gasoline and replaced them with about 200 solidly frozen fish. These were placed on the floor of the Norseman aircraft.

After take off, I said to Gordie, "Open up the heaters, I'm freezing to death."

"Are you crazy," he said, "and have all those fish thaw and slide forward under the pedals! Forget it! We fly back to camp with both the fish and us frozen. After we unload, you can warm up."

I suspect this was a ruse to have me along for company to load and unload. I can't imagine buying fish any fresher. The whole operation was carried out with a completely straight face. Gordie and I got along very well. Later, we enjoyed those big whitefish stuffed with dressing, baked and served in the mess hall, following the rule for Catholics, fish on Friday.

✛ ✛ ✛

One of our early acquaintances was Father Bernard Brown, who was based about forty miles south at Fort Norman. Originally from Buffalo, New York, he had established a parish, built a church and living quarters, found and trained his own dog team and constructed a sleigh and boat with which to carry out his work. He was very much on his own, as his Bishop was based in Chicago.

Hospitality is very important on the frontier. No one can survive without help from others. I first remember Father Brown coming to the hospital for a visit, bringing with him a chunk of moose meat. I suggested he come to the house that evening and we would have it for supper with some vegetables.

The first step was to leave the meat outside for the dogs, as Father Brown was a poor butcher. The second step was for Ruth to go to the mess and draw a roast of beef with all the trimmings. Our third step was the offer of a shower and the chance for him to clean up. We had many delightful evenings like that. I would try to teach him enough anatomy so that he could butcher a carcass properly, rather than just attacking it with an axe. We would argue points of theology, arguments which I would lose. I also tried to teach him enough basic dentistry so that he could cope with the emergencies that landed on his doorstep. We were good for each other.

In the entire western arctic, there were two and one half doctors. Dr. John Callahan at Aklavik, working for the federal government, me at Norman Wells working for Imperial Oil and an inconsistent doctor at Fort Smith. He was the half. I often wondered about his periodic disappearances.

✛ ✛ ✛

Before Ruth and I left Edmonton, I told Dr. Ross Vant, who was the University of Alberta professor of Obstetrics and Gynaecology, that I was going to the Arctic. Having no knowledge of what I was getting into, I asked him if there was anything I could send him from the North. He had always been good to us, providing professional care without charge to a fellow confrere. He was aware of our pathetic financial situation. I appreciated his courtesy and have tried to follow his example of generosity to patients in need throughout my career.

Ross Vant said, "If it isn't too much trouble, I have always wanted a polar bear skin for our cabin at Lake Edith in Jasper Park."

Since I had no idea what I was talking about, I replied, "That shouldn't be any trouble."

Shortly after we got settled, I put the word out for two polar bear skins, one for Dr. Ken Symington in Calgary and one for Dr. Vant. In due time my request was filled. The poor Eskimo who had to hunt, face, kill and skin the two bears sold the skins to the Hudson's Bay Company in Aklavik for $20 and $30, respectively. In their raw frozen state, smelling to high heaven, they were shipped to me at Norman Wells. They were beautiful skins, in their prime. The largest skin was at least nine feet by twelve feet, the other only slightly smaller.

It took me several days to go through all the paper work to export these skins from the Northwest Territories. I needed a license. Luckily for me, one of my many jobs was issuer of fur export licenses so I changed my hats, paid my fee, and issued two export licenses.

I shipped the larger skin to a special tannery in Edmonton for tanning, mounting of head and claws and delivery to Dr. Vant, who was thrilled. Much later he told me it was so large they had to build an extension on his cabin.

The smaller skin was shipped to Dr. Symington in Calgary in the raw state.

When I later got the bill for this undertaking, I wished I had forgotten my bright idea and settled for sending them both something else, particularly when I realized that the man with the bravery, who found and faced the bears, was compensated the least.

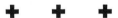

Shortly after we arrived in camp, it became obvious that a lot of money was spent on whiskey and other spirits.

As head of the household, with all of its chauvinistic implications, I announced to anyone interested that Ruth and I didn't drink – in truth we couldn't afford to drink. To my supportive wife, I also added, " . . . but that doesn't mean we aren't going to buy any whiskey."

In the North at that time, and I don't imagine things have changed, whiskey was the lubricant through which to achieve necessary favors. Whiskey at hand, when used with discretion, accomplished both the improbable and the impossible. I note the following example.

About 200 miles further north, Dr. Callahan worked for the feds. He ran a large, busy hospital filled with Indian and Eskimo patients. He was always running short of supplies. Daily telegrams to Ottawa did not alleviate the situation. We had never met, but occasionally we spoke via short-wave radio, when conditions and equipment permitted.

He had run out of Plaster of Paris bandages, essential for building casts. He had an Eskimo lad with a fractured tibia (shin bone). A bottle of whiskey to a pilot friend provided transport to my hospital at Norman

Wells. The fracture was set and a suitable plaster cast made. In a few days, when someone was going to Aklavik, a bottle of whiskey at my end insured transportation of the patient back to where he started.

I never underestimated the power of a bottle of whiskey at hand, especially good whiskey.

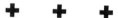

It was Monday and it was cold. During the day, only a glow on the horizon for several hours served as sunshine. The temperature sometimes went down to less than minus forty-five degrees. It made no difference at that point whether one measured in Celsius or Fahrenheit, it was cold.

The doors of the hospital burst open, letting in a tidal wave of cold air. Old Sven, who drove a D-10 Caterpillar tractor, said,

"Doc, you've got to help me, I ran over my teeth."

In his mittens was a collection of bits and pieces of artificial teeth and denture material. The night before he had been drinking, not wisely, but well. His stomach, no doubt his entire gastro-intestinal tract, was rebelling and he had thrown up. In the cold and in his post-alcoholic state, he had run over his dentures with the enormous cleated tracks of his favorite tractor. Most of the pieces were beyond technical recognition, let alone repair. Working outside in such a climate required a large caloric intake, unavailable through a steady diet of soups and slops. This man's survival was at risk. The nearest real dentist and dental labs were in Edmonton. There were no flights out and more importantly, he had no money, having drunk it all.

I had several dental flasks and an odd assortment of unmatched teeth left over from dental school projects. The teeth neither matched in shape, size or color. We collected his bits and pieces, supplemented by my bits and pieces and made for him a pretty sad looking pair of dentures. The teeth were different shapes, different shades, different by any comparative measure. Cosmetically, they were unacceptable. They were by far the worst looking false teeth I have ever seen.

Mechanically we achieved excellent occlusion – they bit well. He could eat anything. As a thing of beauty, however, they failed. No responsible doctor would admit to being their creator. When I finished the final adjustment on the dentures, Sven was thrilled. They fit great, better than his old teeth. These "didn't slide around as much" he told me. He said he could even eat apples and corn-on-the-cob.

"I'll pay you when I get my next pay cheque, even before I buy a bottle," he declared.

There was a problem, however. I did not want to be known as the dentist who created such a monstrosity. I swore Sven to secrecy and told him that in exchange for his silence, I would not charge him. As the company doctor, I could not allow an employee to starve to death.

Sven kept the faith as did I; my only hope was that he eventually replaced them. It is doubtful, as he was only interested in function, but I was also interested in appearance.

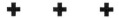

When we initially arrived early in February, the sun was only a faint glow on the horizon. It was only light from 11:45 a.m. until 1:15 p.m., then darkness once again appeared. By late April, the sun was visible in full each day and the welcome rays stayed minutes longer. We kept hearing stories of the phenomenon of "Spring Break-up."

Each spring the camp held a lottery on the "Break-up." There were cash prizes and a historical timetable of previous break-ups was posted. Contestants selected a date and drew for time slots given in ten minute blocks. We selected May 12th, Bill's birthday. We drew the time interval of 7:30 to 7:40 p.m. Official time was calculated by running a wire out to a tripod on the ice. When the wire broke, stopping the clock, a siren sounded. That was the official time of break-up. Our time interval put us in the winner's circle and we collected $360 in cash. A collective groan went up. The crazy teetotaller doctor and his wife had won the grand prize on the break-up of the MacKenzie River. What a disaster!

Usually break-up was followed by a big party with gambling and drinking – by the next morning, the jackpot winnings had been redistributed, everyone had a hang-over and life went on. What a disappointment, a teetotaller won the Jackpot, bah!

The awesome power of the break-up was unimaginable. Great slabs of ice, sixteen feet thick, were thrown up like pieces of cardboard, the force of the push from up the river driving the slabs into the frozen river banks, tearing shrubs up and slicing dirt.

We were accustomed to seeing heavy equipment, such as huge D-10 Caterpillar tractors at work – their strength was puny when compared with Nature. During winter, company operators routinely bulldozed a two-way road across the frozen MacKenzie river to Bear Island. In places the ice measured sixteen to eighteen feet thick. Mother Nature's force during spring break-up tossed large slabs of that road, the size of our house, around like toy blocks.

The Arctic is a land of contrasts. Long, dark, bitterly cold winters suddenly switch at break-up time to spring thaw, which lasts almost two weeks. This quickly leads to summer. Summer, with its very hot days, has almost twenty-four hours of sunlight and no nights. A sudden short autumn, resulting in freeze-up, precedes winter. Your calendar and activities fit the weather.

CHAPTER VI
More Northern Exposure

After winning the Break-up of the MacKenzie sweepstakes, Ruth and I investigated and wondered what we could buy for the camp. Imperial Oil had established off-duty entertainment, which included curling ice, rec centre, games, photo lab, sports equipment and trophies. There was nothing the camp needed.

Once again, Ruth came to the rescue. Together with my head nurse, they came up with a brilliant idea. They would put on a formal tea party for the entire camp. This would be on Sunday, the only day everyone was off.

I said, "Are you girls crazy? Most of these guys don't know the difference between a tea pot and a coffee pot let along a tea cup and a coffee mug."

"You girls want to put on a fancy tea party?" I continued. "You'll be the laughing stock of the entire camp. You're crazy. I don't want to be a part of this ridiculous scheme."

As usual, I totally underestimated these capable, persistent ladies. They didn't need my permission. They didn't even need my help. Their inclusion of me in the conversation had only been a courtesy and I missed it.

The two of them went to work with enthusiasm and both were superb organizers. Ruth wrote to her mother and requested special lace table-cloths, special serving dishes, a silver tea set, candles and silver candle sticks, serviettes and a million other things I didn't understand. She and the pastry chef went to work in the mess kitchen producing great quantities of dainty goodies, finger sandwiches and foods we routinely never saw. This had become a major project.

Ultimately, the company plane arrived with all the packages. The flight engineer said to Ruth, "We have a package for you," as he unloaded the back deck of a pick up truck piled high with fancy foods and special serving dishes.

I was not convinced. I was sure this was a disaster in the making. Both women ignored me. Their attitude was: "Nothing ventured, nothing gained." They worked like Santa's helpers. The date had been set for the following Sunday. Everyone in camp was invited. The menu included dainty sandwiches, petit fours, lemonade, tea and coffee, no booze.

This was my wife's Pink Tea Party for a bunch of refinery workers, roughnecks and Cat drivers and anyone else who cared to come.

When Sunday arrived, I was amazed to see that everyone in camp came. All were cleanly shaved, although some were shaky, many couldn't eat and more than a few coffee cups rattled.

The native kitchen dishwasher put on a clean apron and came out to join us. He complained of having no place to sit and three people immediately stood up. When the fine china serving platters were passed, he took a handful of dainty sandwiches. He had never seen anything like it and obviously found it hard to get enough to eat, based on the number of fine cakes and fancy lobster and crab meat sandwiches he devoured.

The lace tablecloths and silver candle sticks with crystal looked gorgeous. It was a smashing success. My predictions had been entirely wrong. The Pink Tea Party started a trend. Several weeks later, the married couples entertained the singles and so it went round the circle.

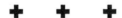

Later in the summer I had a problem. I was approached by a couple of mixed religion and racial backgrounds, who planned to wed in a few weeks. As the Justice of the Peace, I could legally marry them in a civil ceremony. My heart went out to this young couple of mixed backgrounds, neither had much education, yet they seemed so much in love. She had ordered her wedding gown from the Eaton catalog. He had ordered new jeans and cowboy boots from the same catalog. The order was to come by company plane on Friday.

They had approached Father Brown about performing the service and were told that special written permission from his Bishop was required before he could marry them.

As Friday approached, I was unhappy at the thought of marrying this young couple in a civil ceremony. The civil service regulations were pathetic in their brevity, so I tried to expand the ceremony. I had never done a civil marriage and in those days, it was important that they be legally married with the "knot" tied properly. I must be a romantic at heart.

The plane finally arrived, and the wedding gown and the new jeans and boots were aboard. More importantly, the letter from the Bishop giving Father Brown permission to marry this couple was also aboard. My worries about the inadequacies of the service vanished. They were truly and properly married by the priest.

This young couple had insufficient funds to finance air fare to the outside, nor had they enough vacation time from work. However, an old shack on the river bank had been temporarily fixed up as their bridal suite and the rest of the camp allowed them privacy for their two-day honeymoon.

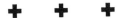

With the warm summer weather, I had constructed a large playpen for Bill at the back of the house. Three four by eight foot sheets of plywood and a surrounding fence gave him an eight by twelve foot play area. Because his cerebral palsy caused spasms of his muscles, he could not walk or run without support. In the machine shop, we built a walker out of electrical conduit pipe, a sling seat and large swivel casters. On this apparatus he got around quickly with no apparent handicap. Ruth had noticed Bill's appetite diminishing, even though he remained well and active.

We were the only people in camp with a child and Ruth was the only person not employed. As shifts changed and the workmen came by the house, they always stopped to talk to Bill and pay him some attention. I'm sure many of them missed their own children.

One day while Ruth was watching, she discovered the reason for Bill's loss of appetite. Many of the workers were rewarding Bill's friendliness with a chocolate bar!

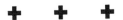

Nick, a welder of Ukrainian origin with an excitable personality, consulted me with a complaint of a recurring right lower abdominal pain. No vomiting, but intermittent nausea and a feeling of uneasiness, particularly when he was bending over in a position he often assumed in his work. Examination findings pointed toward a diagnosis of early appendicitis. At the time, I was short staffed and only had my head nurse and a nurse's aide, hardly the staff needed to undertake major abdominal surgery requiring a general anesthetic.

With luck, I thought, this might settle down. The first step was to give his digestive tract a rest. We prescribed a diet of fluids only. That evening at the mess hall, I saw my patient faithfully sticking to his fluid diet, followed by him picking his teeth with a tooth pick for some time after the meal. I could barely suppress a smile. Old habits are hard to break.

This therapeutic approach lasted forty-eight hours, then he returned with added complaints. His right sided abdominal pain was coming and going with increased severity. Examination showed early abdominal muscle spasm and muscle guarding. Further delay would only make matters worse and increase the risk. This man's muttering appendicitis was becoming more acute with each passing hour.

Performing an appendectomy was within my capabilities and those of the hospital. The problem, however, was anesthetic; attempting this abdominal operation with local anesthetic was not sensible. It would not provide the abdominal relaxation needed and the patient was anxious, not a good combination. I had no one trained, nor available, to give an inhalation general anesthetic such as ether. The only other appropriate choice was a spinal anesthetic. This was adequate for surgical purposes, but it lacked something for an apprehensive patient. I was quite sure he would be upset if he saw me approach his back with a long spinal needle. Intravenous pentothal, at that time, was a fairly new drug. Used with caution, I hoped it would be safe for our purpose. We started an intravenous drip and injected a small dose of pentothal, sufficient to make the patient drowsy. He was then rolled onto his side and a spinal needle inserted at the appropriate level. I injected the correct dose of spinal anesthetic, rolled him back and waited for the anesthetic level to stabilize. He was sufficiently drowsy to be unaware of what I had done.

We scrubbed up again, surgically draped the operative area and entered the abdomen through an incision. My head nurse was the surgical assistant and the scrub nurse. The nurse's aide monitored vital signs at the head of the table. When I found the inflamed appendix, it was worse than I had anticipated. It was just as well we had not waited any longer.

Our patient recovered with no complications. I kept him drowsy until the spinal anesthetic effects were gone. Having an anxious patient awaken with temporarily paralyzed lower limbs was only going to increase his apprehension. He was up and about in several days and back to light work in a few weeks. No further abdominal pain was felt.

Reports concerning employees' health were a requirement of head office in Toronto. The Medical Director teased me about the telegram I sent: "Nick . . . had acute appendicitis, operation successful, post op. condition stable, recovery normal to date." What else was there to say? Still they teased me about the succinctness of my report.

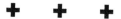

As Bill advanced in age, Ruth and I began having increasing concerns about his slowness in developing proper speech, the spasticity of his motor muscles, his poor sense of balance and his unsteadiness. We knew the Rh factor incompatibility had caused brain damage at birth – only time would allow assessment. Despite our medical backgrounds, as parents we were too emotionally involved to form an impartial and worthwhile opinion.

Winning the Break-up Sweepstakes gave us the necessary funds to fly Ruth and Bill out to Vancouver for a consultation with our old friend Dr. Joe Grant. He had been one of the pediatricians involved at the time of Bill's birth. We had every confidence in his judgement. We had planned to go out together, but once we had made the decision and now had the finances for the trip we couldn't wait, so Ruth and Bill went to Vancouver on their own.

I tried to write an unbiased clinical report to bring Dr. Joe up to date. I sent Ruth and Bill off to Vancouver with hopes and prayers for the future. Deep in my soul, I knew there was no cure, no perfection. At best, maybe we could develop a plan to put this child in an environment where he could cope.

Dr. Joe did his own thorough history, physical examination and assessment of Bill, as I knew he would. When he had finished and completed some phone calls, he said to Ruth, in a most fatherly and professional manner.

"There is a bed for your son in the pediatric wing at Essondale Hospital. There is a taxi downstairs. My advice is to put this child in an environment where he can cope with his life and get help with his problems. You and Jack get your lives back on track and consider adopting a family. Bill cannot function in your world, nor you in his."

We have been forever grateful that this superb clinician was straight-forward and completely honest in his handling of our son's case. His was good advice, clear, concise and included a plan of action. Bill is now in his forties with even more problems. Painful as it was at the time, it was good advice for both Bill and us.

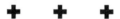

There was a devastating accident in the refinery. It was unusual and unpreventable. Foreman Jim had momentarily taken off his hard hat because his bald pate was itchy. At that precise second a large pulley broke loose, fell two stories and struck Jim on the right side of his head. He dropped to the ground, an unconscious blob of bone, muscle, skin and nerves.

The refinery crew quickly got him on a stretcher and up to the hospital. We made sure there was no obstruction to his breathing, got an intravenous drip going and set about an accurate and detailed examination. The initial examination revealed he was deeply unconscious, however his pupils were equal in size and his vital signs continued to remain stable for the next two hours. His level of consciousness gradually improved. Three hours after the accident, he was awake and cognizant with a full memory. After a further hour, he appeared completely conscious and much like his normal self. To be on the safe side and to reassure myself, I had him carry out a 100 minus 7 test. In this test the patient starts with the mathematical figure of 100 and mentally subtracts 7, gives the sum and so it continues. This test allows a check of recent memory and the patient's ability to do mental arithmetic in a serial fashion. It's a simple exercise, but not always easy to do when your brain has been bruised and shaken by a concussion.

I was beginning to think, rather hope, that we had been fortunate with this accident, but I still had nagging doubts. He seemed bright and alert in the first twenty-four hours and of course he wanted his discharge from hospital. "No sense staying here, eating the company's food and wise-cracking with your pretty nurses," he said. "Let me out, I've got work to do, so turn me loose, please."

There are times the Lord smiles on you and he sends one of His Angels to insert nagging doubts in the back of your head. Some people call it intuition, some call it judgement, some just take all the credit. I call it being looked after by the Man Upstairs.

I was not happy about discharging the patient, so he stayed, despite his protests, complaints, threats and bribery. During the evening he remained stable. Early the next morning, his condition began to deteriorate. He complained of a headache, his jokes lacked luster and often a punch line. His pulse rate had slowed. His reflexes were erratic. He was more and more drowsy, without having received any sedation. Ultimately, he could be aroused, however his level of consciousness was slipping. We were watching the development of a neurosurgical emergency. This man was having a bleed from an injured, probably a torn blood vessel between the membrane under the skull and his brain – a sub-dural hematoma.

Since it was spring break-up there was no serviceable landing strip – no planes in, no planes out – no telephones to the outside world to allow me a vocal consultation with a neurosurgeon. I was the man on the spot!

I went back to the books to read up on anatomy and procedure. I had seen it done in practice a few times, but I had never done the procedure myself. I was not the best trained neurosurgeon in the world, but I was the only surgically trained person available.

While checking the instruments I needed before sterilizing them, a major omission became obvious. The hospital was really not equipped for neurosurgical cases because we did not have a proper drill bit for drilling burr holes in the skull.

I rushed down to the machine shop, I needed a bit and I needed it now! The senior machinist calmed me down and said, "Doc, don't panic, tell me exactly what you need and we can probably make it right now."

"Thanks, Jake," I replied. "I need a 3/8 inch bit with a shallow angle of approximately eighty degrees, so I don't penetrate too deeply when I get through the bone in making my burr holes."

A special bit was quickly manufactured. I rushed back to the hospital, carried out another neurological examination to specifically pin point the site of this man's bleed. We didn't have the diagnostic measures we have today.

Having done my homework, I approached the problem with confidence and a positive outlook. We did a scalp shave, marked the position of the planned incision with a ballpoint pen (felt pens were not available), injected local anaesthetic, incised, raised the scalp flap, reflected the periosteum covering the bone. No matter how many times I have surgically uncovered bone, I am always impressed with the whiteness of this hard living tissue, it virtually glistens. Now to drill the burr hole. It worked well, the drill was sharp. Now to carefully examine that underlying membrane. It looked dark, almost black, suggesting a blood clot underneath. Cautiously I held up the dura (the membrane) with my thumb forceps and carefully nicked the membrane all the way through with a scalpel. The blood was dark and clotted, confirming the diagnosis, a sub-dural hematoma.

I tried not to congratulate myself yet and just kept going. I sucked out the blood clot to relieve the pressure on the brain tissue and ensure that there was no fresh bleeding. Once the wound was dry, I got out, suturing each layer as we replaced it.

The patient made a rapid recovery. The operation appeared to be harder on the surgeon than the patient.

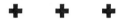

Our Arctic living experiences were unique. We had made some wonderful friends. In my opinion, Imperial Oil treated their employees with compassion and understanding.

In the spring, we were part of an important new experiment. Freight costs to ship vegetables were about one dollar per pound, expensive in those days. Could we grow fresh vegetables for the camp? If we could it would be great – no more cans! The company had the local soil analyzed, supplied the lacking minerals and fertilizer and we started the interesting experiment. The camp had a proper garden with a knowledgeable gardener, and even an entomologist with imported bees and worms. Interested residents were given a plot, seeds, fertilizer, rakes and other tools.

As described earlier, due to the ground being permanently frozen, water lines and accompanying steam lines ran above ground. The water was heated to prevent it from freezing, consequently the ground was also heated. We were approaching long days of sunshine. The expression "throw in the seeds and jump back" was almost true. Germination and growth were unbelievably rapid. We were able to grow above-ground crops. Some below-ground crops were hampered by perma-frost which, even in summer, kept the ground frozen twelve to fifteen inches below the surface.

The gardener was able to grow an assortment of vegetables. Some of the novice gardeners placed tomato plants in the heated soil where steam lines ran adjacent to water lines. To people accustomed to eating from cans, miracles happened almost before their eyes. The tomatoes were lush, red, juicy and delicious. I am not a gardener, but I do enjoy fresh vegetables.

This experiment provided an amazing quantity of food for the camp. Apart from fish, no local animals were available for meat. Caribou were further north. The barren landscape did not support large quantities of wildlife suitable to feed the employees of our camp. Our gardening experiment was to learn what we could grow and harvest to support the camp. Fresh tomatoes and lettuce were great for morale. Almost as good for morale as when the Imperial Oil plane had space in their cargo hold to fly in fresh milk.

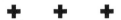

Shortly after spring break-up, the RCAF arrived and set up their own camp. This consisted of a squadron of three DC-3s with ground support crew. They were carrying out the first official aerial mapping survey of Canada. Prior to arriving in Norman Wells and while attached to the Toronto head office of Imperial Oil, I had contacted Air Commodore Corbett, at his request. He had a proposition for me. If I provided medical services to the squadron based in Norman Wells, he would provide a nursing Sister. We would supply her quarters and rations and she would move out with the squadron when they left. This would give me an extra nursing staff member during the summer when we were busy with the extra traffic and people on the MacKenzie river.

The Commodore and I made a deal. No paperwork, no consultants, a straightforward deal, a handshake from one officer to another. I had just one stipulation, I wanted someone capable. He was as good as his word. He sent me Flight Lieutenant Ella Mannix, an excellent Nursing Sister and a lovely person with lots of personality. Just the type to fit into our routine.

In this day of complex deals, it is difficult to conceive a deal as simple. That's no doubt why it worked so well.

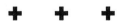

Early one morning, I received a telephone call from the local signal corps detachment. They had monitored a transmission from their Fort Smith station. The message was vague: ". . .someone in labor for many hours. . .Doctor away paying treaty money. . .HELP!" They repeatedly tried to raise Fort Smith, no success. There was no answer. The RCMP were at our air strip refuelling their plane and offered us a lift. Shirley and I grabbed what we might need and accepted their offer.

During the flight we contacted each district. As we flew over Fort Norman, the district nurse came on the air for a consultation about a fellow with a severe fracture-dislocation of the ankle. She wanted advice about reducing the dislocation. The district nurses were a special breed. They had to be medically self-sufficient, serving as both doctor and nurse. They did a magnificent job under the most trying circumstances. We carried out the consultation until we flew outside radio range.

After flying about two hours, we landed on a dirt strip across the river from Fort Smith. We were met and boated across the river to the community. Amazingly, this community had a two story hospital run by the Catholic Sisters. Yes, there was mother in labor. Yes, the doctor was away paying treaty money, but he could be reached if necessary. Why had we come so far when there was no emergency? Who had sent the emergency message?

We paid the signal corps a visit and found the young father-to-be who had hit the panic button. We were the farthest away, so had no chance of confirming the message. Whereas others within radio range had had the opportunity to ask questions and assess the situation, we hadn't, so had responded, thinking the worst.

The Sisters kindly made arrangements with the wife of the R.C.M.P. officer for a bed for Shirley and they put me up at the hospital. The next morning, I begged a ride home with an R.C.A.F. transport aircraft, whose crew kindly diverted to pick us up. The signalman was chastised. In the future he would get permission to broadcast the equivalent of an S.O.S. in the western Arctic.

Our return trip was made in a DC-3 and we were wedged between bags and cartons of freight. There were no windows and no heat. I would not do that again, because it left the people at the refinery without coverage had there been an explosion or fire.

I heard later that the couple had a son, normally developed and good, healthy weight. How could I stay angry?

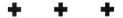

There is a lot of traffic on the MacKenzie River during the summer, including weird aircraft. One day an old Sikorsky flying boat landed, flopped is probably more accurate, on the river and struggled to the dock. We were accustomed to all kinds of aircraft, but this was a museum piece. We presumed they wanted to refuel. In truth, this was a magician and his wife from Chicago, bringing their magic show to the Arctic. They entertained us that evening. It was not an enthusiastic audience, the natives were scared out of their wits and the camp members were bored. In keeping with the hospitality of the North, we provided them with lodging and food.

The next morning they tried to take off. They tried unsuccessfully, many times. When the expert mechanics in camp took a look, we were amazed that they had survived this far up the MacKenzie. The boat part of the aircraft was awash with at least four hundred gallons of water. Their bilge pump didn't work and the hull was full of holes. The magician knew little about aircraft maintenance and his wife had reason to worry. The least we could do was carry out the basic repairs to make them somewhat airworthy.

Once the weight of the water was removed, the aircraft hull patched and the craft refuelled, they tried again. No go. We had another aircraft taxi cross-ways in front to create waves, giving the flying boat enough lift to get up on the step. Eventually it became airborne and gradually climbed to a height of about two hundred feet. We heard that they leap-frogged north to Fort Good Hope, on to Arctic Red River and eventually to Aklavik where they sold the engine. The hull sank and they returned to their home in Chicago never to venture north again.

During the summer, when the sun shines twenty to twenty-four hours a day, the pilots literally go without sleep. Many times their only sleep is a quick snooze on the wing while their plane is being loaded or unloaded, refuelling they did themselves. They were, for the most part, careful pilots, but regulations sometimes were stretched. It was not unusual for them to fly triple overloaded. The engine would strain and the runway distance would be used to its limit and beyond. The collective intake of breath of those watching seemed to provide that extra lift at the last minute, then there was a collective sigh.

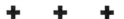

Late one afternoon, a pontoon-equipped Norseman came over the hospital at an extremely low height of about twenty feet. I was in the lab looking out the window and could easily count the rivets on the bottom of the pontoons. I knew the pilot had amorous intentions for one of my nursing staff. "Buzzing" the hospital was not the way, however, to tell her that he was back from a trip. When I went to supper at the mess that night, he knew I was looking for him. I did not appreciate having my hospital buzzed; it was a hazardous, juvenile trick. He was well aware of my feelings. Before I had a chance to open my mouth in anger, he apologized and gave an explanation. He was flying back from Aklavik against a stiff head-wind, triple overloaded and had been watching the gas gauge red light tell him he had been out of fuel for several minutes. He took the shortest route possible, one over the hospital roof allowing him to land on the water. As he landed, he ran out of gas and the engine died. He had to paddle to the dock. I accepted his apology.

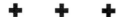

In mid October, 1949, we left the North. The number of employees in camp had dropped to less than fifty; a doctor was no longer needed, so I was posted to Imperial Oil's head office in Toronto. My duties were pre-employment and annual physical examinations. Unfortunately, any condition requiring treatment had to be referred elsewhere. I received excellent training in industrial and occupational medicine, but found this was not the challenge I was looking for and following some discussion, Imperial Oil and I ended our working relationship. They were good to me and I appreciated working for them, but the time to leave had arrived. My departure was carried out on excellent terms.

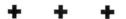

On our return to civilization, in the east, we purchased a 1949 two-door Ford at Port Credit, just outside of Toronto, where it was cheapest. Driving our new car back into the city, we were terrified of the traffic on Yonge Street and had to stop at a cafe to regain our confidence. We were only used to three or four trucks on a single road and this was a brand new car, ours!!

During a few weekends of travelling to see our friends and relatives, Ruth and I discussed our future plans. We didn't have enough money to continue my education as a maxillofacial surgeon. That meant moving to the U.S.A. Meanwhile, the field of plastic surgery was clarifying its boundaries, burns and cosmetic surgery and in large industrial centres, hand reconstruction and repairs. The latter interested me, but no immediate training posts were available. I knew I did not have the personality to devote my life to cosmetic surgery. It became obvious that wartime reconstructive surgery and peace-time cosmetic surgery both sprang from different needs; the former from a desire for function and the latter from a worship of beauty and perfection.

At that stage of medical specialization, the big three were Internal Medicine, General Surgery and Obstetrics-Gynecology. The specialty of Eye, Ear, Nose and Throat was an orphan off in the corner. Subsequent specialties have all been built upon those four bases and are off-shoots of developments in each of those areas.

The more I though about specializing, the clearer the answer – I really wanted to look after people and families – Family Practice. At that time it was called General Practice, an old-fashioned G.P. That was my true ambition.

The next questions was "Where?" The obvious answer was in the West. We travelled back to the wonderful "Marriott Hotel," where the board and lodging were free and we had an endless supply of love and concern. "Are we ever going to get this young couple launched on their career?" Father Marriott would ask with a smile.

We had always believed that we would set up practice in Vancouver. At the end of November, we went out for a look. The fog was so thick, the seagulls were sitting on first-storey window ledges because they couldn't see where to go. Everything was wet and rusty and the sky was always overcast. We had come out of the land of twenty-four hour sunshine. This was too much. After three days, we drove back to Calgary. The sunshine welcomed us and we stayed.

CHAPTER VII
Family Practice

We covered most of southern Alberta in our survey of possible practice sites and kept coming back to Calgary as if it were a homing beacon. The Marriotts lived on Frontenac Avenue in southwest Calgary. At the bottom of the hill was an intersection (14th Street and 17th Avenue S.W.) where the street car turned. On the four corners were a bank, a jewelry store, a drug store (Crooks) and a confectionary run by Jimmie Condon. Jimmie owned the building, which went between 16th and 17th Avenues on the west side of 14th street.

Next to his confectionary was an unrented space, previously a beauty parlor. We struck a deal and in the process started a life-long friendship.

Jimmie had been in business in Calgary for years and had all the contacts to help me convert the rental space into a first-rate medical office. K.P. Neilsen's crew put up partitions of wood panelling for eight feet, with two feet of glass on top, creating ten-foot walls. Originally designed as a store, the heating consisted of a single large register in the floor and the ceilings were at least fifteen feet from the floor. The front entrance was a door beside a large display window. In this we hung a large gold leaf sign: "Dr. John R. Ibberson, Physician and Surgeon," at the height most easily seen from the bus, which stopped directly in front of the office. Most of the other physicians in Calgary thought I was crazy to establish an office in the suburbs. They were all downtown in the Greyhound building, the Calgary Associate Clinic or the C.P.R. Clinic. Because of Jimmie's help and the position of our "shingle," we never went a day without seeing patients.

In retrospect, this was one of the initial family practice offices in the suburbs. It seemed logical to me that if one wanted to practice medicine for families, one had to go where the families were. I noted that mothers didn't feel they had to dress the kids up when brought into the office, as compared with taking them downtown. This was an advantage for me, because if they weren't gussied up, I didn't have to do any de-gussie-ing before examining them.

Since we were between families, Ruth worked in the office as my nurse. She was outstanding; quick, knowledgeable, excellent with kids and their mothers and she knew how to keep "The Boss" on track. I learned more practical pediatrics from her than I had from any textbook.

Jimmie's corner, as it was called, was a good place to start and Jimmie was very helpful. Jimmie Condon was a true gentleman, Greek by birth, he adopted Calgary, worked hard in the food and candy business, and became a legend, due to his support of junior athletics. One of his last acts was to import and donate two large marble statues to the University of Calgary medical school.

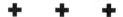

Each year Jimmie would sponsor the immigration of several Greek families to Calgary. Initially, they all lived in two large houses which Jimmie owned. Many became my patients. Most of the wives became pregnant and came to my office. Not one spoke English and I have no knowledge of Greek. When looking after these ladies, I often tried to put myself in their place. If I were pregnant and attending a doctor in Greece, with no knowledge of the Greek language or customs and knowing nothing of the hospital facilities, I would have been terrified. But not these ladies. I carried out pre-natal examinations and educated them, mainly in pantomime. Sometimes the mime became so hilarious that everyone had a giggle, but somehow we still managed to communicate. I drew pictures, I mimed, I flipped through a Greek-English dictionary, and despite my lack of knowledge of Greek sentence structure or tenses, we managed.

As these pre-natal office calls went on, so did the pregnancies, through to delivery. In those days, the fathers were not allowed in the delivery room, which was just as well. Can you imagine the excitement and confusion? I was having enough trouble just handling the mothers. I don't recall any of the deliveries being a problem, but then starting with a young, healthy mother always helps.

Those were special ladies, some a little more excitable than others, but all special nonetheless. I remember one afternoon receiving a frantic call. One of the two-and-a-half year old boys was trying to be very grown up by standing at the toilet to pass water. In mid-stream, the seat came crashing down onto his. . .need I say more. What chaos, two or three languages in mid-air! She didn't believe that "it" wouldn't fall off; a tragedy to his manhood. She rushed him into the office; "it" was bruised and bloodied. However, The Man Upstairs knew what he was doing when he designed these organs; they have an admirable blood supply and heal very quickly and there are seldom any complications.

As time went on, Jimmie's two houses were home to many families, each with numerous small children. When I made a house-call, I usually saw four or five sick children. I was often not sure who their mothers were, because the women who acquired English skills were out working. Most of the husbands started work as cooks for Kentucky Fried Chicken.

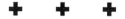

With time, this led to interesting financial complications. This was going on about the time we doctors introduced the Alberta Medical Insurance Plan called Medical Services Incorporated (MSI).

In the beginning, patients were identified by name, not by number. When these people immigrated to Canada their names were Petropolous. As they Canadianized, however, some became Petros, some Polous, while some stayed with Petropolous. As this transition occurred, they often did not let us know and our patient cards became more and more inaccurate, almost useless. At the point of total chaos, I contacted the medical director of MSI and we tried to reach a conciliation. I was only sure of one thing, they owed me a certain amount of money generated by services to the entire Petropolous clan, but exactly which one or ones was open to question.

The final solution required a trip to Edmonton. The medical director put all his information from the computer on the table and I did likewise with my office cards. We discussed it, we went out for a drink and came up with a figure we could both live with. Shortly thereafter, the system changed to numbers to identify patients, no doubt caused by me.

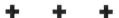

About the same time that we had established the office, we found a suite in an older home several blocks from the office corner. The owner, a widower, lived downstairs while we took the upstairs. We had a bedroom, a living room (previously a bedroom), a bathroom, a kitchen (previously a bedroom), a front hall, and a flight of stairs. We had little furniture, a bed, a trilight and a large cabinet radio.

To establish a credit rating, we purchased a double bed from the Bay and a small electric stove from Eaton, agreeing to pay off these debts over three months. After we had cooked supper, we ate it with our backs to the wall sitting on the floor in the living room listening to the console radio. After doing the dishes, we read the paper in the same living room in the same position. At bed time we took the trilight into the bedroom, and when it switched off the day was over. After we had paid for the bed and stove, we splurged and bought a kitchen table and four kitchen chairs. Later we purchased a second-hand ice box and refinished it.

On occasion, we invited Ruth's mom and dad for dinner. Ruth's dad would puff up the stairs, enjoy his eldest daughter's cooking, then comment, "Well, I guess we had better go up to our place to find some chairs to sit in after that wonderful supper! We will take our car because yours doesn't have a back seat."

The Ford two-door we bought in Ontario was a travelling salesman's model, with only a deck in the back (for sample cases). It was their cheapest model.

I'm afraid that this type of hospitality went on for some time, but I'm sure they enjoyed it as much as we did. Now that I'm older, I can see things through their eyes. If I was near the Purity Flour Mills, my father-in-law insisted the staff fill up the doctor's car from the gas pump for the trucks (I know it went on his account). They always had a garden at the mill and he would insist that I take home a 100 lb. sack of potatoes and 100 lbs. of flour.

When I said, "Dad, how can just Ruth and I eat one hundred pounds of potatoes or use one hundred pounds of flour?" He said: "Hell, it's not worth packing anything smaller!" He would have a fit with the small packages of today. He was a salesman and a miller through and through, one of God's special gentlemen. We quickly developed a deep relationship.

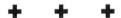

One morning, after finishing rounds at the hospital, I was up on a ladder, dressed in overalls, cleaning the large front window outside the office. A young man walked up and said, "Is the doctor in? I would like to see him." I replied from my perch on the ladder, "He just called from the hospital and is on his way. Why don't you go in and wait? He will be along shortly." I finished the window and slipped around to the back, unpeeled my overalls, put on a white jacket and walked up to the reception room to the young patient.

"Can I help you? I'm Dr. Ibberson."

He did a double take and said, "Didn't I just talk to you outside cleaning the window?"

I couldn't help myself as I replied, "Must have been my twin brother, he helps with the maintenance."

When you're just starting a practice, never discourage a potential patient, no matter what you have to say!

Establishing a practice brings increased financial indebtedness, and thence the need for a life insurance program. My examiner was Dr. Robert Francis, Sr. (the senior was to differentiate him from his son, James, a surgeon who practiced with him).

When Dr. Francis Sr. finished with my examination, I asked, "How does a young practitioner start a practice in Calgary?"

"Well, young fellow," he replied, "if I were you, I would go to the Holy Cross Hospital first thing in the morning and drink coffee in the doctors' room just off the operating room. Get to know the doctors, and maybe someone will need a surgical assistant or someone to make a house call for them. The next morning I would go to the General Hospital and do the same thing. So your intentions are not too obvious."

This was excellent advice and it worked. I got to know Dr. Gordon Townsend, an outstanding orthopedic surgeon. He knew I had training in his discipline and used me as a surgical assistant and general helper for the first few years. The work was much appreciated.

There were a total of ninety doctors in Calgary at that time. They were all hospitable and we were invited to the pre-Christmas cocktail parties and made to feel welcome.

Several older doctors would often phone in the middle of the night and say: "Young fellow, Miss or Missus so-and-so is at the General or the Holy Cross ready for delivery. I am terribly tired, would you please take care of her?"

In those days, the maternity fee was $35 for everything. If the doctor got paid, I would get $15 for doing the delivery. If he got nothing, so did I.

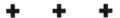

The delivery had gone smoothly, a little boy. He was having difficulty getting his first breath due to some obstructing mucus in his airway. Initial suction was not successful so we laid him on the edge of the table so I could put in a laryngoscope and suction more effectively under direct vision. In those days, the case room nursing uniform had a square-cut neckline. When the girls were leaning forward, such as this nurse was doing to restrain the baby for me, the exposure was delightful. With me putting down a laryngoscope and a suction tube at the head end, reflexes occurred. He emptied his bladder. A thin yellow stream flowed right down "the Great Divide."

I was devastated. The nurse didn't comment. She just held the baby until I got him breathing. I then said to her, "I'm sorry about that accident. If you want to slip out and change, I can manage here."

With a flip of her head, she said, "He didn't hit a thing, I'll just blot dry. I'm fine, really."

Great women to work with. There are no pretenses and nothing fazed them. Getting the baby breathing was the only important issue.

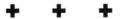

Obstetrics has always been a fascinating part of medicine for me. No matter how many babies I deliver, it is still a miracle. Stories abound of thrills and tragedies in this area. I have always tried to teach interns that this is a special time for a woman. She invites you to share a unique part of her life. She never forgets the doctor who delivered her first baby.

Another memory involves an attractive, athletic tennis champion in the third trimester of her pregnancy. One morning as I was driving between the General Hospital and the Children's Hospital, this lady, shopping at Safeway, was approached by a wandering radio reporter. He learned that she held the ladies' singles tennis championship and asked her if she was going to defend her title in the coming matches. She was using all kinds of hints to explain why she was not going to defend her title. Her pregnancy was quite obvious. Apparently this reporter was blind and dumb.

At her next pre-natal visit she filled me in on the details. In her words: "I kept shoving 'it' in his face and he still didn't get it."

There was no way, at that stage of her pregnancy, she could have run up to the net and stopped. It is a treat to look after women with a sense of humor. She ultimately delivered and was a great mom.

Usually maternity is a happy time in medicine since most mothers are young, vibrant and healthy. The catastrophes, although few in number, are still terrifyingly clear, even after forty-five years of practice. These cases leave scars that never heal, thank goodness, because from these scars we learn and teach our lessons to others.

One of my biggest fears was the death of a mother. This devastation never occurred in approximately 3000 deliveries. We had some close calls but never a fatality. My alternate fear was losing the life of a baby. This has happened. It is crushing in its grief to the mother and father, whether it is in utero pre-partum, or at the time of delivery or shortly thereafter. It is also crushing to the doctor.

One of the painful recollections is of a wonderful lady I had attended during her initial pregnancy. A routine normal pregnancy with a normal cephalic (head first) full term birth weighing 8 lb. 2 oz. The baby thrived.

Subsequently she again became pregnant. The pre-partum course was normal. Her weight gain was well within normal limits. As she approached term, we determined this was a breech (buttocks first) presentation. Such a presentation can be straightforward or complicated in the extreme. With a past history of her pelvis being able to pass a normal 8 lb. 2 oz. head first baby we didn't anticipate problems. Since the second pregnancy was a breech presentation I had re-x-rayed her pelvis to check pelvic measurements. They were average sized, they seemed adequate on pre-partum assessment coupled with her history to allow delivery of her second child.

She went into labor and we monitored her progress carefully; she was doing well and making good progress. That afternoon I had to go to court as an expert witness. Momentarily, I thought about leaving this maternity case for the intern to deliver, then one of God's Angels sitting on my shoulder poked me and said, "You know this is a breech and that crises can develop."

Having received this warning and it being very good advice, I contacted one of the top obstetrical specialists in the city.

"Doug, I don't think this lady is going to have any problems. She is in good condition, her past history is on the chart. Last time she delivered an 8 lb. 2 oz. baby in record time. My concern is that with this delivery, she is presenting as a breech. We both know problems can occur. Please keep an eye on her for me while I am in court. I will see you as soon as I'm off the witness stand. Thanks."

I did not get out of court until 5 p.m. I rushed over to the case room and met Doug coming out of the delivery room. He looked ghastly and spent beyond recovery. He was pale and his voice was a whisper when he said, "I couldn't deliver the baby's head. The baby died." Then he visibly shuddered. "The mother is fine, she knows. Go and talk to her. I'm going to shower, change and go home. Sorry this did not turn out as we expected."

He looked absolutely exhausted.

Before I went to see the mother, I called Doug's wife, and said, "Don't ask questions. When he gets home have a drink ready for him. If he wants to talk he will; if not don't push. Maybe tomorrow or next week he will tell you. He has just been through a most devastating experience. The baby died but the mother survived."

Then I changed my clothes into operating overalls to go to the delivery room to see my patient and her husband. What a remarkable couple, they were trying to comfort me. After the catastrophe they had suffered, their compassion was extended to me.

The next day an autopsy revealed this child had weighed 9 lb. 4 oz. The additional eighteen ounces and the resultant increase in head diameter was just enough to prevent delivery and cause the tragedy, just enough to make the difference between success and failure. In this day and age, a scan would indicate a caesarian section.

All the additional details of this case are history, but there is a pleasant ending to this agonizing tale. Several years later this marvellous lady again attended me for maternity care. This time we did not even consider giving her a trial of labor; we delivered her by Caesarean section. Although I don't recall whether it was a boy or girl, I do remember it was a normal, healthy child, what the parents and I had hoped.

How can I explain what goes through a doctor's mind in handling such a case; the responsibilities, the trust the parents grant you as their physician? You assist at a miracle and try your best. If a tragedy occurs, your soul is torn and heals with a scar.

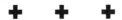

Shortly after starting practice on 14th Street and 17th Avenue S.W., I rejoined the armed forces, 403 Squadron R.C.A.F. (Reserve). This was a fighter squadron which flew Mustangs. In flight, the side profile of a Mustang suggested a pregnant aircraft, due to the bulging air scoop below the propeller. There was nothing pregnant about their performance.

As the senior flight medical officer (Sr. M.O.), I did the pre-enlistment medicals and was responsible for medical service on Thursday evenings and Sundays.

Most members of the squadron were veterans, like myself, although my service had been in the army. The newly enlisted recruits were keen on learning all the skills required for aircraft maintenance and repair and, in the case of pilots, the training and qualifications leading to a pilot's license. We had the old experienced hands and the new eager beavers.

One amusing incident pops into my head. A newly qualified pilot, more enthusiastic than cautious, was brought to the M.I.R. (Medical Inspection Room) with a complaint of an earache. When questioned about what happened, he admitted bringing the aircraft down in a vertical dive and going too fast, allowing the aircraft position to get beyond vertical. Then in a desperate effort to avoid ploughing into the ground head first, he had done a 180 degree roll and flattened out about 200 feet parallel to the ground, popping every rivet in the wings and tail and pulling back the wings by three inches. I believe the mechanics pulled out the radio, navigation and oxygen equipment and junked the airframe wings and tail.

After the C.O. (Commanding Officer) had finished his blistering attack, which the pilot may not have heard, he was brought to me. Examination revealed a severe hemorrhage in both middle ears and a rupture of both ear drums.

Our conversation was short and terse. "Pilot Officer, as you came hurtling down from 40 000 feet, full bore, did you not swallow, as you have been taught, to equalize the pressure inside and outside your ear drums?" In a quivering voice he whispered, "Eh, what did you say? Doc I don't think I even breathed, let alone swallowed. I was so scared when I lost control of that baby. Honest to gawd, I thought I was going to dive into the ground head first. Why can't I hear so good?" I smiled. Maybe it was just as well he hadn't heard everything the C.O. had said as he peeled blistering strip after blistering strip off him. The C.O., a veteran Wing Commander, was upset – no, he was mad as hell. On top of which he had to "write off" an aircraft he could not replace and explain it to his superior officers.

I only had to deal with a pilot with traumatic bilateral hemorrhagic middle ear problems and ruptured ear drums. If the C.O. hadn't already grounded him, I would have, for medical reasons.

+   +   +

That unfortunate incident was the precursor to a real tragedy. One Sunday afternoon, as I finished my flight surgeons duties and headed for home, I was aware that all aircraft had not returned from the day's exercises. As I walked into the house, planning to take my visiting mother and family out for a Sunday night dinner, the phone rang. It was the C.O. – the Wing Commander – and he had just received a report that a Mustang had ploughed into a steep hill off Highway 22 near Priddis. I asked to be transferred to my Sergeant in the M.I.R. and told him to be sure to bring a ground sheet in the ambulance. Bring a stretcher O.K., but be sure to bring a ground sheet. He was young and had no experience recovering bodies, or pieces thereof, from crash sites.

Knowing the pilot, an experienced squadron leader with two overseas war tours, I had to suspect the reason for the crash was anoxia (failure of oxygen equipment) rather than pilot error.

Flying in the reserve on Sunday and Thursday reverted the pilot's status to active service when on duty. If this was an anoxia-caused tragedy, he was entitled to full service coverage. I knew he was married, and as I recalled they had three small children – a new born, a two year old and four and a half year old. To prove anoxia, I needed spinal cord and brain tissue samples stored in liquid nitrogen. This had to be shipped in a vacuum bottle to the Air Force pathology service in Ottawa.

The intimate details of digging out a pilot who has gone into a hillside at 300 m.p.h. you need not have described – the ground sheet was a requirement.

Later at the Col. Belcher Hospital, the D.V.A. (Department of Veterans Affairs) hospital, I called the pathologist and asked him to come down so we could obtain the tissue samples I needed, preserve them in liquid nitrogen and ship them to Ottawa to prove that this experienced pilot had died of anoxia.

My anger mounted to heights I didn't know existed as he said he would not come down and do an autopsy because he had an uncomfortable emotional reaction when he did an autopsy on a battered body. There was a large red ball of emotional retorts whistling down the telephone line in his direction, starting with, "Emotional reaction! What the hell do you think I have just been through. Digging a close personal friend out of a cockpit buried twenty feet into the hillside. I'm fighting for pension for his widow and education for his children! If you won't come down to your pathology department, I will do it myself. At all costs, I am sending fresh specimens to Ottawa to prove this was anoxia. Tomorrow the tissue will have aged and won't show anoxia. Good night."

My reaction in hanging up the phone was like slamming the door. I hoped the glass would break. It didn't. I cannot ever remember being so mad, before or since.

We got the specimens and proved it was a crash caused by oxygen equipment failure and the pilot becoming unconscious at 45 000 feet. He had slumped forward over the controls and dove straight into the ground, at full throttle.

After driving out to his home, one of those small houses on 34th Avenue, near the Marda Theatre, and talking to his wife, I hoped she was able to hold their lives together. The evening ended as I got home late, no supper, no appetite.

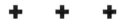

On an amusing note, the Air Force had difficulty paying me. The paper trail had to start with my discharge from the R.C.A.M.C. (Royal Canadian Army Medical Corps) in July, 1946. They could not seem to prove that I had actually been discharged from the army. Therefore, they could not initiate pay documentation in the R.C.A.F. This was not a pressing issue for a few months, but I had taken this R.C.A.F. job to help pay some bills generated by my starting a practice. We really did need the money. It was not until I suggested that since I had not been discharged, then I would take my back pay from the army at the rank of Major. This would cover the period from 1946 until the present (this was in 1952). The paper trail proved I had been on active service with the army, so I had a point.

Eventually, after more than one year in the R.C.A.F., the paymaster said, "Come to pay parade tonight, Doc. We can pay you!"

I received one year's pay in cash! I was scooping up money, shoving it into my pockets. The fellows had a crap game ready to relieve me of my dollar bills. I was too scared, too much in debt to do anything except go home and dump it all on the bed for Ruth to see. I can't remember how much, but it was quite a few hundred dollars which we needed desperately. The sight of cash is more impressive than a cheque, something to remember when you are bargaining.

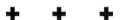

Several months after we started the office, we underwent all the interviews, supplied all the required references of good character and a summary of medical history required of prospective parents wishing to adopt a child. It was time to start a family again. We had not been successful with the traditional method – fortunately, another alternative was available.

Can you imagine the excitement when one Friday afternoon, early in December, our social worker phoned the office and said: "We have this little boy in the newborn nursery at the Holy Cross Hospital. Would you like to look at him and see if he will do as your adopted son?"

See if he will do?! Social workers have the strangest way of asking questions. We whistled patients through the office as quickly as we could. It seemed to take forever. They all kept asking about this and that and I wanted out of there! Eventually we got over to the newborn nursery at the Holy Cross.

He was lean. No, he was skinny. He was a wiggler and he had rubbed a good deal of his very dark hair off his head and some skin off his heels. We fell completely in love with this fourteen day old child. Ruth wanted to take him home right then. He was handsome, but he looked a little worn and hungry. Emotionally, we knew it was right. Even so, how do you tell a social worker you don't want "that one," you'll wait for "the next?" That choice is not allowed when you get children the traditional way.

We had nothing for babies. We had given it all away during the hiatus. We were resourceful, however, and got cracking that night. The next morning we picked him up. I said to Ruth, "Where is he going to sleep? We gave all the baby furniture away."

"In a bottom drawer," she said.

"But all my shirts are there," I replied.

"Not anymore. We have a baby."

Then it suddenly dawned on me that this lady to whom I was talking was also my office nurse. "What am I going to do for an office nurse come Monday?" I asked.

"I don't know. It's not my problem, I just became a mother. You solve it."

She was very excited and I could understand why. It had been a long wait. We named our son John Richard.

The upstairs of that crazy old house was not well heated. There was no insulation in the walls, only shavings in the attic. John's birthday was November 23, 1950. By the time we got him home, the December weather was cold. The nail heads on the closets were ringed with frost. The only room consistently warm was the bathroom, so he lived there for the first few months, in a bassinette in the bathtub. It didn't damage his psyche, and it kept him from freezing to death.

Everyone in the large Marriott clan was thrilled with our adopted son and none more than Ruth's mother and father. They remembered the previous heartbreaks and like us they were thrilled about the future. Still, I felt sorry for my own mother. With her inflexible eastern up-bringing, her feeling was that he was not in her bloodline and therefore he was unacceptable. It was a pity that these feelings blocked a normal grandmother's affection for a newborn. Unfortunately, she struggled with these feelings all her life. I know she wished things were different. The contrast was even more marked by the total and unconditional acceptance and love expressed by Ruth's mother, now called Gran.

With this young fellow on board, life settled into a family routine, something we had missed. Our on-file order for a refrigerator was finally filled. No more dripping in the front hall and up the stairs by the iceman. We even got a $25 rebate for our old ice-box and soon we were able to buy a washing machine.

My practice was growing. Each day I was busier, becoming better known to the community. I was on the active medical staff of the hospitals, teaching Infectious Diseases to the student nurses in the Holy Cross Hospital, working shifts in the Emergency at the General Hospital, and becoming involved in the Red Cross Children's Hospital (later to be the Alberta Children's Hospital).

CHAPTER VIII
Houses, Kids and Cowboys

One evening shortly after we had gone to bed, Ruth complained of a hot electrical smell. She had complained of this before, and I had checked and looked at everything and found nothing abnormal. This evening I leaped out of bed into the dark hall connecting all our rooms. A little blue flame was making its way up the wallpaper from the electrical wire on the far side of the meter.

This house had been wired long after it was built and in many areas the wire ran on the surface of the walls, held away by porcelain insulators. This was the source of the hot electrical smell, a fire in the making in the hall at the top of the staircase. Had the fire erupted in force, we would not have been able to get down the stairs, there being no other way to escape in this two story house. The windows were too small to allow passage of a body – we would have been trapped.

I cut the power by removing two fuses, but the problem of hot wire was in the circuit on the other side of the meter and I couldn't cut that power without interfering with the circuit from the power in the back lane.

I called the fire department and calmly reported a potential fire. They came back in their straightforward manner and said: "Doc, what do you mean a potential fire? Either it's burning or it isn't."

I repeated my explanation. Their solution was to send someone from the City electrical department.

The repairman arrived about 2 a.m. "Did I have a flashlight?" Yes. "Did I have a ladder?" In this house, such trips meant going downstairs, out the front door, down the sidewalk, in a side door, downstairs to the basement and returning the same way. I brought up the ladder. "Did I have a screwdriver?" For what type of screw? Same trip repeated. "Did I have sandpaper?" Again, the trip. In all I made five trips getting this fellow tools and equipment with which to do the job. Obviously this was a consultation; all I was getting was the brains and experience, no labor. After he cleaned all the connections, he thought it was safe until morning. All night, we slept with one eye and both noses open.

Several weeks later I received a bill from the City Electrical Department for $25 for the night visit of our electrician. In those days, I received $12.50 for a middle of the night house call and I had to bring my own tools!

The next morning, three fire trucks arrived. The fireman inspected the suite and house, then informed the landlord who lived downstairs that the house was condemned unless an extensive list of improvements were carried out. He was quite elderly, a cardiac cripple and not interested in rebuilding the house from the inside out. Our days were numbered.

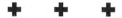

We had been looking at houses for some time and wondering if we would ever be able to afford one, but there was a discrepancy between our wants and our resources. We continued looking, only now with more urgency. We contacted a builder and discovered some available serviced land in south Mount Royal. We could not afford to buy a house, but we could afford to build. With temporary cash flow assistance from Ruth's mom and dad, we took the plunge, purchased the lot and started drawing plans. We thought we knew which lot was ours, until the morning Charlie Priddy's men started to dig the hole for the foundation. Charlie ran down to City Hall for a permit. A couple driving by stopped, ran over and wanted to know what we were doing digging a hole on their lot!

Charlie returned with news the real estate companies and the city had mixed up the titles of the lots. We were building a two story house on what we thought was a lower piece of land, they were building a bungalow on higher property. In the end it worked out to everyone's satisfaction.

We built a lovely two storied house with a central hall plan. The excavation was dug two feet deeper than usual, giving us a high ceilinged basement with plenty of clear space – a good location for children to play and adequate room for a workshop. Two thirds of the basement had painted walls and floor, protectors on the lights and was separated from the workshop by chicken coop wire fencing. I could see and talk to the children yet they were isolated from the woodworking machinery. I didn't have worries about our own children; the mystery of the tools was gone with explanation and the noise they made. My concern was with visiting small friends. As a further safety measure all tools were wired through circuit breakers I could turn off as I left the shop.

I had grown up with a workshop and acquired an understanding of working wood. When we lived in the upstairs suite, Ruth had saved her fifty cent pieces and bought me a Delta table saw for Christmas. She could not afford the motor, that came later. The good quality table saw she got me is still in use today, some forty-eight years later.

Our new home had no furniture so the shop produced the children's bedroom furniture. Made of clear birch most of it is still in use in the family today. In addition to the regular items I made them each a personal desk and matching book cases, which I'm sure encouraged them to be readers.

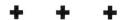

Shortly after we adopted John, we resubmitted all the papers, repeated the interviews and gathered the required affidavits to recommence the adoption process. This resulted in our again attending the new born nursery early in 1953 to bring home our ten day old beautiful daughter, who we named Nancy Ruth.

We often used the services of an older widowed farm lady as a babysitter. She thought John was perfect; in her opinion we would never be lucky enough to adopt another baby as wonderful. When we got home with our new daughter, Mrs. Mac. at first sight fell in love with this child and said, "You can't tell me anything different, those two parents got together again. She is just as cute as John." There was no point in bringing up facts, her mind was made up. Mrs. Mac. had that wonderful mother's capacity to love little people.

Meanwhile, the Marriotts had sold their large family home on Frontenac Avenue and bought a new bungalow about two blocks from our new home on 12th Street. The intervening distance became a well worn path for little people, their parents and their grand-parents.

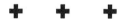

Nineteen-fifty-one was a difficult, emotionally depressing year. I lost a brother-in-law of whom I was fond and a father-in-law, whom I worshipped.

Ruth's oldest brother, Jack, a navy veteran, worked in Vancouver for Canada Safeway's accounts department. A routine physical examination disclosed a testicular tumor which proved malignant. The prognosis was poor. He had been in Safeway's head office in Calgary and wanted to return to Vancouver to finalize his affairs while his wife remained in Calgary. Ruth and I could not accept him doing this solo. Although we could not afford it, we arranged for Gran to look after John, allowing Ruth to accompany her brother on his final trip.

During that two week period, I am sure Gran mentally relived Jack's early childhood through our John. A special relationship developed between John and Gran, possibly because he was adopted, possibly because he came along at a very special time, no one knows.

At the same time Jack Marriott returned to Calgary for admission to the Holy Cross Hospital, Ruth's dad was also admitted as a patient with heart problems. Suddenly John got very pale and was admitted for investigation and a transfusion. We had all three in the Holy at one time.

Jack died on March 31, 1951. Mr. Marriott had increasing cardiac problems, which ended peacefully on the morning of August 22, 1951. He was 72. He was wonderful gentleman who had overcome a lifetime of gargantuan problems. Early in life he worked for Bausch and Lomb, the lens makers in Rochester, N.Y., U.S.A. and Hamilton, Ont. Multiple middle ear infections, due to his being a championship swimmer, before the development of antibiotics, had left scarring which resulted in deafness.

A spot on the lung (tuberculosis) at an early age meant he was sent West for a cure. There, he acquired the infection of typhoid and spent an entire winter being nursed in a tent city in Brandon. His spiking high temperature was beneficial in arresting the tuberculosis and neither infection surfaced again. He became my surrogate father and set an example to strive for when doing business, living life and interacting with people.

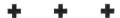

One of my early cases was a two year old boy. This youngster had been seated on the upper basement stairs, watching his mother do the washing in the basement. He fell under the hand rail to the concrete floor, sustaining a severe skull fracture and head injury. He was admitted to the Holy Cross Hospital, deeply unconscious but stable. We watched his progress carefully and he seemed to be gradually improving. On the second day, his mother was most anxious to have him home, but I did not feel comfortable about discharging him. I asked my general surgeon friend, Dr. Jim Francis, to see him in consultation. In those days, we did not have a neurosurgeon practicing in Calgary. Most of the neurosurgical accidents seemed to end up in Jim's or my hands. We had each received some training in this specialty, but much preferred, when we could, sending these cases to Dr. Guy Morton, a trained neurosurgeon in Edmonton.

Jim Francis saw my patient early that evening. I was in the operating room repairing a hand that had come too close to a table saw blade. In those days, we could talk to each other through an open operating room door. Bureaucracy and a fear of spreading germs has now eliminated hall-to-operating room consultations.

Jim was not pleased with his examination findings. Since I had seen the child in the morning, his level of unconsciousness had deepened. There was evidence suggesting increasing pressure inside his head. Jim thought the child's condition sufficiently stable to safely move him to the General Hospital, where we kept what neurosurgical instruments we had.

One flap of bone of the fracture was becoming depressed and was putting pressure on the brain. We transferred him to the General, planning to operate that same evening. We arranged for one of the anaesthetists to be brought in to closely observe his vital signs and to maintain an adequate airway. As the child was deeply unconscious, we did not need an anaesthetic as we started the operation. When we got through the soft tissue and slowly started to elevate the depressed bone flap, the child began to regain consciousness. Dr. Clarke, our anaesthetist, gradually put him into a controlled sleep with anaesthetic gases. We carefully elevated the bone flap and suctioned out the blood clot. Our little patient was improving and we were quite pleased.

As we inserted the last scalp skin suture, tragedy struck. Suddenly there was no pulse, no breathing, no heart beat, no response to anything we did to resuscitate him. The anaesthetist could not revive him. One moment he was doing well, the next moment he was dead. We were thunderstruck. We had no idea how this tragedy had occurred. The bottom to his and our world just dropped out.

As I pulled off my gloves and operating room gown, my thoughts went to the parents waiting in a small room at the end of a long corridor outside the operating room. What could I say to them? This child was the same age as my own son. Just days before, this child had been sitting on the cellar steps watching his mother do laundry and now he was dead. She would no longer be the recipient of his constant stream of questions, nor hear his giggle at something appealing, nor see his wonderment over new discoveries. What a terrible thing to have to tell those trusting, loving people and what could I tell them, except the truth?

Just then, Jim Francis turned and quietly said, "Would you like me to come down with you when you talk to the parents?" If a special bond had not existed between us before, it certainly came into existence then. It was a long walk down the corridor.

I don't remember exactly what I said to the parents. I know it broke their hearts. Shortly thereafter, the father, who worked for Massey-Harris farm equipment, was posted to head office in eastern Canada. They came into my office to thank me. I have never felt so completely inadequate.

They gave me their trust; they left their son, their most cherished possession, in my hands for repair; unfortunately, my skills were insufficient and he died. These are the times in this profession that push you to the wall and drive you to learn more. I shared their tears.

Some months after this tragedy, Dr. C.W. Taylor established his practice in neurosurgery. Jim and I welcomed him with open arms. We were glad to have a neurosurgeon in town. We reviewed the case of our young patient with him, as well as other cases. I was able to write the boy's parents and explain that we could not have saved his life even with the most expert and advanced facilities. He had suffered a severe brain-stem injury from which there was no recovery, in those days.

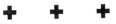

One of my early patients in the Foothills country was a Gary Cooper type of working cowboy, lean and taciturn. He silently limped into the first examining room, sat and gingerly eased off his boot and sock. His great toe was flattened, the nail completely black. You could almost see it thumping.

"What happened, Herman?" I asked.

"My favorite horse stepped on it."

"Well, let's fix it."

Using an old fashioned trick, I heated the straightened end of a paper clip to a red hot temperature. With this, a painless hole is quickly made in the nail. The trapped blood and serum squirted out. It stopped thumping. The hole was covered with a gauze dressing.

As I turned to leave the examining room, Herman crossed his legs and carefully eased off the other boot and sock. His great toe was dislocated.

"Oh, my gosh, how come?" I asked

"'Cause I kicked him for stepping on me!"

One quick expert pull reduced the dislocation and his foot looked normal.

Curiosity made me ask, "How can this happen to someone around horses all his life?"

"I forgot I was in my socks! Thanks Doc."

With a wave and a smile, he swung into his pickup and was gone.

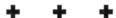

The Lucky Strike convenience store, west of the city limits, was a landmark for doctors making house calls. Patients would phone for help and every doctor would use the Lucky Strike store location as a reference point.

I acquired a family of mother, father and four small children who lived in a rundown house one long muddy mile from the Lucky Strike store.

The father's occupation, apart from procreating the species, was uncertain. They did have a sign in the window saying, "Tatooing done here." I did not have sufficient skin to allow payment of their account. Telephone calls for help would never come to the office. They always came to my home at about 11 or 11:30 at night, delivered by one of the small children calling from the Lucky Store. All you received was a request, such as: "Mum wants you to come out now, to see Joey."

"What's the matter with Joey?"

"I don't know, she wants you to come out now, tonight. Will ya?"

"Can't you tell me anything about Joey? Does he have a fever? Is he throwing up? Has he been sick for long?"

"I dunno, mother says come now."

These conversations were unsatisfactory. The only solution was to get dressed, drive out to the Lucky Strike store and plough through the mud, in the dark with no street lights, for another mile, slop through more mud and snow drifts to their shack. Once there, I often discovered there was no emergency.

These calls went on for several years, and during this time, we carried mother through several pregnancies, never being paid for any services rendered.

The family was well known to the doctors who practiced in town. Most of us did more than our share of charity work. Talk in the doctors' coffee room at the hospital revealed that once Dr. John Maxwell had seen this father peel off a five dollar bill, but before Dr. Maxwell could get it, mother, large as she was, executed a superb end run and plucked the five dollars from her husband's hand and deposited it in her ample bosom. At least Dr. Maxwell had seen money. None of the rest of us had been so fortunate.

One night, after I had again carried this lady through a confinement and delivered her baby, another call came from one of the children.

"Mother wants you to come out tonight and see the baby."

Again I ploughed through mud and entered their humble dirty messy home. The conversation, as I recall, went something like this:

"Mrs. . . . what is the problem with the babe?"

"Doctor, I called you out because I think it is time to change the baby's formula. I think it needs to be stronger."

Of course, she wasn't breast feeding. I examined the child, biting my tongue and revised the infant formula. Then, in the sweetest voice I could muster asked, "Now, Mrs. . . . is there anything else I can do while I am here? Are they any other medical problems? Are all the other children fine?"

Everything seemed under control. This gave me the opportunity I had hoped for, no, prayed for. There were no other medical problems.

"Mrs. . . ., I have been very good about providing my services and receiving no remuneration. I have done my share. There are presently no problems, therefore I am not abandoning you or your family. The time has come for you to seek services from another physician. You have free choice of doctors, as I have free choice of patients. I do not choose to continue our medical relationship." This was said with clarity and firmness.

She looked at me aghast and said:

"What do you mean, Doc? You ain't goin' to come out when I call you, no more? I gotta find someone new and train them?"

I replied as sweetly and as courteously as possible. "That is exactly what I mean. Bless you, Good Night."

Thus ended my relationship with that family. It was time for someone else to share their free medical problems. This was long before welfare systems. Many doctors of my vintage could share unending stories of a similar nature.

Of course, the Lucky Strike store is no longer there. The roads are now paved and doing a house call on out the Old Banff Coach Road is a delight enhanced by the beautiful scenery.

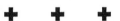

In the early hours of the morning, the insistent ringing of the telephone summoned me from the depths of slumber. It was the maternity case room – "Mrs. . . . has just arrived and we need you now."

Years of habit and established reflexes take over in the absence of organized thought. Leap out of bed, throw on some clothes, rush to the car and head for the hospital. At the first stop light, I momentarily went back to sleep, came to and thought, which hospital called? I remember it was Mrs. . . . she would probably go the Holy Cross, I'm sure. Rushed there, hurried into the doctors' change room, slid into a green scrub suit and ran to the labor rooms. There sat the head nurse and one of the staff nurses, charting and knitting. After I finished chastising them for not paying attention when a patient was in labor, they sweetly informed me, "We didn't call you. We have no one in labor, doctor." Oops!

Rushed back to the doctors' locker room and quickly changed back into street clothes. Drove as quickly as I could to the Calgary General Hospital and ran to the case room to be greeted by, "What took you so long to get here?"

There was barely time to scrub for the delivery, then I confessed my stupidity to the nurses. They, of course, were wide awake and full of quick remarks, such as, "What would you do, doctor, if there were four hospitals doing maternity? Make rounds and then drive the child to kindergarten?" That was the only time I recall going to the wrong hospital.

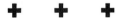

Many years ago, long before the development of anti-depressant medications, one of my patients, after each delivery, would develop a severe post partum depression. The only effective therapy in those days was electro-convulsive shock treatment. In her case, a single shock was usually effective.

After the delivery of one of her multiple offspring, she did not slip into her usual post partum depression. I did not understand this, so curiosity made me ask, "Mrs. . . . with each delivery in the past, we have had to deal with a post partum depression. Not this time. Why not?"

She answered, "As a matter of fact doctor, I was developing a depression after the baby was born. I was starting to feel quite down. Then I was doing the wash in the basement and the floor was wet and the plug to the machine was frayed. When I plugged in the machine, I got a frightful shock. It really quite scared me. Strangely, after that shock I started to feel less down, less depressed."

I had my answer – self administered shock therapy. Not recommended, quite hazardous, but in her case effective.

As she grew older her disease process declared itself more clearly, and she was diagnosed as a manic-depressive. She copes quite well on a regulated daily dose of Lithium.

CHAPTER IX
Home, Work and Play

I seldom touched home when our small children were up during those busy years and that resulted in some memorable happenings, sparked by son John.

In Grade one, during an exercise known as News Period, he started a rumor. John's news was, "Daddy doesn't live at home anymore. He lives at the General Hospital and when he isn't too busy he comes home to see us."

A word of explanation: at that time I was handling a heavy obstetrical case load, usually 25-30 deliveries a month and also working shifts in emergency, as well as running a busy full practice. This was in the days before we had interns to lighten the load. John's statement was not inaccurate, it was phrased to lead to false conclusions.

Fortunately, the teacher knew my wife and saw the humor. A phone call resulted in the following exchange: "If I didn't know better, I would surmise you two were heading for a divorce."

Ruth said, "I haven't seen enough of him lately to even talk about it!"

Even so, we heard some interesting rumors in the neighborhood.

The things that happen in doctor's families are probably no different than the happenings in everyone's family. John was the one with a million questions, usually early in the morning when my mind was in idle, not in gear. One Sunday morning, when I was in the middle of doing my hospital rounds, I was paged for a phone call. It was Ruth.

"John has been out playing with his friends and came in and said, 'Hey Mom, what's a picnic?' I don't know what you have planned for the rest of the day. I just ordered a taxi and I'm taking John and Nancy and we're picking up Gran for picnic in Riley Park. If you want any lunch, you know where we will be. It's ridiculous that the boy doesn't know what a picnic is!" Click. End of telephone call. As usual, Ruth was absolutely right. Our own son should know what a picnic is and she was going to set things right. Having a busy husband was no excuse.

Being blessed with a capable, loving wife has made my life easier, more interesting and has allowed me the privilege of doing the many things I have. We had a great picnic in a beautiful park in the centre of the city.

John was always a questioner. He had learned something about boxing and how to duck. He insisted on asking his mother to box with him when she was trying to prepare supper.

She said, "There isn't enough room in the kitchen and you will get hurt."

"No I won't. Try to hit me, so I can show you how I learned to duck."

Sure enough, one duck and the edge of the kitchen counter split open his eyebrow. There was blood everywhere.

When I arrived home ten minutes later, a pale, subdued boy was on the chesterfield with an ice bag on his eye. It was obvious this gaping wound needed stitches.

We made a modified bed in the back seat of the station wagon and set off for the General Hospital. After a few blocks, this faint voice from the back seat said, "Do you think I'm going to make it?"

Trying desperately not to laugh, I replied, "Oh, yes, I think you'll make it. We haven't lost any of these types of cases, so far."

With a leap he was in the front seat, color already returning to his face. As we drove along Macleod Trail, I said, "You know, your old friend Dr. Francis is out of town and so is your friend Dr. Pow. What would you think about me sewing you up?"

There was a long period of silence while he considered this. Finally, with a completely straight face, he said, "Dad, have you ever done one of these cases before?" That was the day I decided, he was a survivor.

We reached the hospital and completed the necessary repairs to his eyebrow. He was as good as gold. The nurses in emergency made a fuss over him. How could they do otherwise?

I slipped upstairs to see a newly admitted patient while they showed John a stomach pump and other gadgets in emergency. Curiosity is a great asset.

I don't know when John learned to type. He seemed to be born with the ability. I'm sure he was typing in Grade one or two. In those days, I had an old Smith-Corona portable machine pensioned off from the office. John took to that machine and they became inseparable; he even took it with him in the station wagon. Wherever he went, he was busy typing a story or a play for the man at the Banff Park gate or his grandmother.

Once we were driving along and I got caught up in doing my fatherly thing and said, "John, why don't you look out at the beautiful scenery, the mountains and the trees?"

John replied, "What's so great about a tree? We've got lots of them." As usual, my comments were premature to a six year old.

His ability to create stories and plays, and ultimately music, persisted into his adult years. One time, I asked him how he did this. His childhood reply was the clearest explanation of the creative process I have ever heard.

"It's easy Dad," he said, "You just get an idea and you unfold it." Out of the mouths of babes...he never did explain where all those ideas came from.

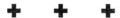

A family with nine offspring were special for one reason: I had delivered eight of the children. The mother ran the home with a special touch, lovingly and efficiently. If she needed me, she called early in the morning knowing my schedule almost as well as my wife, and when she called it was not for one sick child, but usually two or more. Making a house call was something like adding another hospital to my morning rounds.

Going through the living room, I stopped to correct the chords Jim was playing for his music lesson. Going through the kitchen, I was aware one of the younger girls was washing and an older taller sister was drying and putting away. Force of habit, as an old army medical officer who had inspected many kitchens, made me drag two fingers through the dish water to check it's temperature – tepid at best. Tiny hands don't tolerate the scalding hot water needed to destroy germs. After attending the two patients upstairs, I left.

Several days later, the mother was in the office and I remarked on my kitchen inspection, commenting that since the family had experienced several episodes of gastro-enteritis, consideration should be given to acquiring a dishwasher to sterilize the dishes and break the cycle of infections.

Without hesitation, this lady of action placed one of my prescription pads in front of me with the comment, "You have your own pen." Reacting with reflex action, I wrote, One Dishwasher, please, and signed it. We laughed about it and I forgot it.

That evening her husband phoned me and commented, "Ibberson, you are so bright and quick! You know there is no point installing a standard dishwasher for family this size. I have a commercial restaurant model being delivered next Tuesday. Since you are so smart with a comeback, you can come up and do the electrical wiring while I do the plumbing. On second thought, bring a bottle of Scotch, if it works the first time, we can christen it."

I went, I wired, we tried it, it worked – so we christened it!

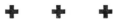

One afternoon my classmate, Dr. Joe Moriarty, called and asked if I had had an unusual number of mothers bringing in six and seven year old boys for examination concerning possible undescended testicles and associated hernias.

The testicle grows from tissue near the kidney and only descends into its normal position in the scrotum shortly before birth. A small number of testicles grow down there shortly after birth, even a smaller number may require surgical intervention to find their new home.

Joe ran a family practice downtown. My practice was in the suburbs. When I thought about it, Joe's assessment had been correct. A lot of mothers had recently brought in their sons for specific examination with a query about undescended testicles. I had the perfect treatment centre, however, a four foot circular hot air register in the floor of the first examining room. I could stand the little fellow on the register and easily demonstrate to mom that his testicle descended to its proper resting place when warm.

Joe was a straightforward, ethical caring practitioner. Secretly, I was pleased to be one step ahead of him as this didn't happen very often.

Joe said, "You don't suppose we are having an epidemic of undescended testicles on our hands, do you? I've never thought of it as being contagious."

"Joe, have you stopped to consider who the school doctor is?" I could not resist the temptation. "I interned with her in Vancouver. She is tall, angular and has very cold hands. When she examines these little guys, with her ice cold hands, their testicles skitter back up inside to a warm place. Wouldn't yours?"

"Oh, my Gawd! I forgot all about that. It makes a lot of sense. I wondered if we were having an epidemic which didn't make sense."

I could hardly suggest that my confrere wear mittens when she was examining these little fellows. The next year her duties in the public health system changed. Amazingly the "epidemic" ceased.

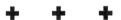

I know a Head Nurse on a Children's ward, Sam by nickname, who is skilled with little patients. One such patient was my friend Susan. We had been pals since her birth. In Susan's mind that was a long time, in reality about six and a half years. We had been through many experiences together, starting with her delivery and proceeding through colic, colds, scrapes and bruises and a broken arm when she fell off the monkey bars.

Susan was hospitalized for removal of her tonsils and adenoids, bothersome things that keep getting infected and re-infected throughout each winter. With each throat infection, her middle ears became involved resulting in her becoming temporarily deaf. These infections gave her a wretched time. Her mother and I had made a decision. The removal of her tonsils and adenoids was booked for early the next morning. During my late evening hospital rounds I saw her for a pre-operative check.

"Hi, Susan. How are things? You are not lost in that big bed, are you? Did you have supper, what did you have?"

"Things are O.K., Doctor Jack, I guess. This sure is a big bed, but it is O.K. I kinda miss my bed at home. We had macaroni and cheese for supper. What did you have?"

"I haven't been home for supper, yet. I came in to see you after I finished at the office. Tomorrow morning is the big day, the day we get rid of those tonsils. Do you remember what I told you was going to happen?"

"Yeah, I remember, I think. We have one more sleep, then in the morning I don't get any breakfast, I don't drink anything and they come for me with a cart with big wheels, I put on a funny hat and go to the operating room. Another doctor puts me to sleep and you fix my tonsils. Then I wake up and I can have some ice cream. Isn't that right?"

"Susan, you remembered all the things we talked about, perfectly. Gee, you're a smart kid and pretty too."

"Yeah, but I've got these two loose teeth. They won't keep me from having ice cream, will they? Dad says we may have to tie a string around them and hook them up to the door knob. They wouldn't do that, would they? He is teasing, isn't he?"

"Susan, let me see your loose teeth, please. They sure are loose, aren't they. I don't think we will have to tie a string around them to the door knob. I may have to fix them when you are asleep. They shouldn't stop you from eating ice cream."

She had two quite loose baby teeth. These worried me. If they became loose during her recovery from the general anaesthetic, she might inhale them into her windpipe or lung. A minor inconvenience then became a major emergency.

The next morning in the operating room, she underwent the induction phase of the general anaesthetic without incident. Before starting her tonsillectomy, I removed the loose teeth with a forcep and asked the circulating nurse to wash them and tape them onto Susan's hospital chart.

After finishing the surgery, as I was writing her post operative orders, I added an additional order. "Please have the Tooth-Fairy call."

Early the next morning, while starting rounds on the children's ward, I asked this little people's head nurse, Samantha:

"What do I owe the Tooth Fairy?"

"Four dollars," she said,

"Four dollars! You must be kidding. FOUR DOLLARS! When I was a kid it was a nickel, maybe under special circumstances a dime, even a quarter if there was a lot of blood, pain and suffering. I know we have inflation, but how can it be FOUR DOLLARS?"

She replied sweetly, with a completely straight face, "It's one dollar for each tooth and a two dollar contribution for the Flat Footed Senior Nurses Fund."

"You are joking?"

"No, I'm not. That is the rule on the ward. You know that. You have done hundreds of tonsil cases."

"Yeah, but not that many with loose teeth that I removed and then asked the tooth fairy to call. She is an expensive fairy!"

"Doctor, you know all fairies are expensive."

Just then we arrived at Susan's bed.

"Well, young lady, how are you after your big operation? You look a little pale. Are you drinking?"

"I'm O.K., I think. I don't have my loose teeth. They are out and the tooth fairy came. Look."

Clutched in her small hand were two one dollar bills. She was proud of her special reward. Obviously I had to reimburse the tooth fairy, at the going rate.

"When can I have my ice cream?" she asked. "Remember you promised."

"Susan, you can have your ice cream a little later today. Let's get your stomach settled before we feed it ice cream. I will come by later this morning to see you and decide about sending you home."

As we continued seeing other little patients, I said to Sam, "I guess I am on the hook to the tooth fairy."

"Yes, you are," she replied. "You wrote the order so don't try to evade your obligation."

That sweet smile and straight face almost convinced me that a Senior Nurses Flat Footed Fund existed. In addition to my two dollar debt to the tooth fairy, I had so overreacted that I felt obligated to provided a box of chocolates for the nurses. As Head Nurse, Samantha demurely accepted and I was treated to a smile and a wink. What wonderful ladies to have as co-workers.

A week later, Susan and her mother came to the office for her post operative assessment. Her throat was healing quickly. Mother told me a most intriguing tale.

"After Susie came home from hospital, she bounced back quickly. I was making sandwiches for lunch and had a bottle of dill pickles open.

Susie asked if she could have a pickle. I couldn't imagine anything worse after having your tonsils out, but I recalled you saying to feed her anything she wants. I remembered how you told me your own daughter ate soda crackers endlessly after having her tonsils out, so I gave her a pickle. She made a face and in one big gulp it was gone. From that moment on, Susan ate everything."

"Wow! I'm not sure I would have recommended that, but these little people are a breed unto themselves and they often know what they can handle, if we listen to them."

Susan and I had many other adventures together, as she grew up.

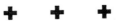

I recall another of my patients, Karen, who had a thyroid tumor. She and her family had been patients for some time. In the process of doing a complete physical examination, I found an enlargement of the lower part of her thyroid gland. This enlargement had to be removed to accurately determine if the growth was malignant and to relieve the pressure on her wind-pipe.

Many important structures exist in the neck – this was major surgery. The recurrent laryngeal nerve passes along the surface and sometimes in the tissue of the lower pole of the thyroid gland and is often damaged or severed in doing a radical resection of the thyroid. That is what we had to do, since the rapid pathological assessment of the tissue we initially removed during surgery was reported to be malignant.

Both Jim Francis and I had warned Karen about this. If the nerve is damaged or cut, partial paralysis of the affected vocal chord occurs. The patient is left with a husky voice and cannot shout or yell. The result is permanent.

We completed the surgery; to completely remove all the malignant tissue we had to sacrifice the recurrent laryngeal nerve. I waited in the recovery room until she was partially awake.

"Speak to me Karen, I want to check your voice." I said. It sounded pretty low. I wasn't sure. It could be the result of the endotracheal tube the anaesthetist put down her throat to maintain her airway. We had to wait.

Early the next morning while making rounds, I could hardly wait to see Karen. She was sitting up against three pillows, neck swathed in dry gauze dressing, no bleeding and she had had a stable night.

"How's the voice, Karen?" I asked.

"A little low," she croaked back to me.

"I'm sorry," I said, "it is a little husky. We had to cut the nerve to remove all the tumor. I'm sure we got all the tumor out and the lymph glands were clear. We'll know better in a few days when the pathologists give us a complete report. I'm really sorry about your voice, but we were out to save your life."

She looked at me with her big brown eyes. You develop a special rapport with your patients when you carry them through a number of pregnancies and deliver their babies.

"My voice isn't husky. It's sexy," she said. She was serious. No feeling sorry for herself.

During the next few post-operative days, we discussed this in more detail. She told me how she had devised a solution to handle her four small children. With a voice that could not yell or shout, she would get a police whistle and a wooden spoon.

She had her follow-ups in my office and the cancer clinic for some years until her husband was posted to Toronto. After quite a few years, she came to my office for a re-check. She still had her big brown eyes and her sexy voice.

During her many years in Toronto, she had follow-ups in the Princess Margaret Hospital, their facility for cancer treatment, radiation and chemotherapy. When asked about her follow-ups, she said she had started in the hands of a young, intense clinician who had just completed his fellowship examinations and was full of the latest statistics. She was teasing me with her big brown eyes and her sexy voice as she said, "You didn't tell me all the terrible statistics about this disease spreading and the real possibility of my becoming an angel."

My only reply was, "Well Karen, at your age, with your family of small children and with us watching you, I figured it was statistical information you didn't need in your bag of worries. When you told me your voice wasn't husky, just sexy, I knew you were a survivor and told your husband so. Here you are, years later, children grown and you are doing fine. It was my job to worry about those statistics, not yours."

She gave me a kiss on the cheek and a giggle. That's a pretty good fringe benefit!

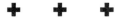

The water is Calgary is naturally hard. We had one of the city's first water softeners installed in our home. It caused problems. Men came up to look at it and did things, but it still caused problems. Eventually, they coated the brine tank with thick, black tar-like material. This caused even more problems. Ruth found black specks throughout the wash. These had to be removed by hand – a very time consuming process. One day, Ruth had had it and burst into action.

The company name on the machine read the Oshkosh Water Softening Company, Brandon, Manitoba. She was so angry she called them long distance.

"Hello, Oshkosh Water Softening, may I help you?"

"Yes, this is Mrs. Ibberson, in Calgary. May I speak to the president?"

"I'm sorry, he is out. Is there anyone else you might speak to?"

"I want to speak to someone who can make a decision – today – and I don't want to be put off."

"Yes, I will connect you to our sales manager."

There was a pause, during which time the switchboard operator probably passed along the message: "I've got an angry customer on the line."

"Hello, I understand you are having a problem, may I help?"

"This is Mrs. Ibberson in Calgary. I'm sure you've never heard of me and now I feel a little foolish calling you, but I'm annoyed."

"Oh yes, Mrs. Ibberson, I know you've been having problems with your water softener. I'm sorry."

"The real reason I called is to tell you people you can have the machine. I'm fed up with the fixing. I would like it out of here, today!"

"Please, leave it with me. I will do something about it today, I promise."

That evening, we went out. When we got home about midnight, Inga, the babysitter, was distraught.

"There is a man in the basement. He insisted on coming in. He is banging on the pipes," she told us.

I went downstairs. He was banging on the pipes all right. He was putting in a new water softener. A company engineer, he had driven non-stop from Saskatoon at the insistence of the sales manager. He had not eaten since lunch. I took off my coat and started to work along with him. As we were finishing, he said, "Have you got any white enamel to touch up these pipes? I think this lady may be pretty fussy." I agreed and got the enamel.

As Ruth was cooking him a steak, at about 3 a.m., she was somewhat embarrassed. "If you are not getting satisfaction from a company," she said, "what should you do?"

He was a red head, very polite and with a piece of steak poised on his fork, looked at her with a twinkle and replied, "Lady, you did it."

The new water softener worked perfectly. Ruth phoned the sales manager to report satisfaction and to express her thanks.

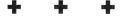

Nancy and John were always competitive. She was two years and two months younger and anxious to do everything John could do. She would be sweet and cooperative until she coaxed him into teaching her something, then tease him relentlessly until she needed to learn something else.

Even then John was a born teacher. A desk or table, proper books and Nancy must give him her undivided attention. She could read long before she went to school, but would not do so until the first day of Grade One. She said, "Your are not supposed to read until you are in the first grade."

Strange how these ideas sneak into little people's minds. Even today, Nancy is more of a private person than other members of the family.

Nancy's mind usually goes at breakneck speed. As a little Brownie, she came home one day in tears and great sobs. We couldn't make head or tail out of it. Finally Ruth figured it out. Nancy wanted to earn her "Homemaker's Badge." To do this she had to clean up after supper and wash the dishes by hand. How could she possibly do this when we had a dishwasher?

Ruth mopped up the tears and pointed out that we didn't have to use the dishwasher. The relief was like someone turning on a light bulb. There was a solution to this catastrophic problem. She could earn her badge.

We had bacon and eggs for supper that night and Nancy, up to her elbows in soap suds, earned her coveted badge.

Another time, the Brownie troop was camping in the foothills. When she came home, she told us they had discovered a wonderful idea for keeping warm. If you put rocks around the camp fire then put them in your sleeping bag, it made everything toasty warm. I had trouble listening to this with a straight face. Each generation discovers for themselves.

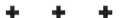

Over my years in practice, I have had few staff. Originally on 14th street and 17th avenue, I had a young lady whom I thought was excellent, until I was an emergency admission to the Calgary General Hospital with kidney stones. It was during this time we learned she had been robbing us blind.

I was en route to the operating room for exploratory surgery when my accountant informed me that the sizeable amount of cash I thought was in the office account had dwindled to a few hundred dollars. She proved to be a real professional thief. It seems that everyone in private practice eventually joins the light-fingered club. My initiation was four figure expensive.

At the time of my emergency surgery, we had a young lady bank employee living with us, named Verna. In those days, before telephone answering services, we not only needed a sitter for the children, we also needed one for night and maternity calls.

Ruth got home late one evening after visiting me in the hospital and Verna said someone had delivered a Christmas present, which she had put in the 'fridge.

Ruth opened the refrigerator door and there sat a beautiful turkey, complete with head and feet. From the leg dangled a business card and a Merry Christmas sticker which read: "Courtesy of McInnis and Holloway," one of the local undertakers.

I was very sick and the prognosis was not good. They had just told Ruth that I might not make it. The first thought that popped into her mind, instead of gratitude, was, "I wonder if they want to exchange one old bird for another?" To be fair, she was pretty tired, as she had lived through quite a few long worrisome days and nights.

In the days when this was the custom, there were fewer doctors. To whom would funeral directors send Christmas greetings and gifts? Still, I must admit, if you got a nice gift, it made you wonder about your practice batting average.

I never enquired of another physician what he received, nor did anyone enquire of me. I guess it's the thought that counts. They tell me it was a delicious bird.

While I was lying in the hospital, spiking an up and down temperature due to infection and not expected to survive, my wife and my accountant had to deal with the police, change the locks and hire a new girl. They hired an eighteen year old business school graduate named Sheila. I worried about a girl of that tender age working in a doctor's office amid the tragic and seamier aspects of life which were seen daily. Eighteen must have been a more tender age years ago; Sheila was a dandy.

Although she was just eighteen, Sheila was mature. She was well trained and we clicked right away. She was with me for about seven years, married our postman and became a mother. Her life has been interesting and tragic.

Sheila was a great help during the creative problems when the medical profession of Alberta initiated Medical Services Incorporated (M.S.I.). She put up with me rushing off to emergency College Council meetings. She juggled patients, handled the Greeks and put up with my dictation often given as I was eating lunch, smoking a cigarette and/or driving to Edmonton. She put up with a lot and made sense of it. She ran a busy office smoothly. She needed her youth to put up with what I was loading on her.

She handled all the correspondence, summary of minutes, emergency meetings and all the activity generated as the Canadian College of

General Practice was born. We needed separate filing cabinets for the para-medical organizational work in which I was involved. As I cast my mind back to those busy days, I thank Sheila, she made it possible.

Sheila was replaced by Barbara, who worked with me in the Academy Building until she met a Mountie.

Many years ago when T.V. dinners were a new item, John created an interesting experience. Late in the afternoon of a busy day, Barbara got a call from John. He had put two T.V. dinners in the oven to heat for supper and smoke was now pouring out the oven exhaust.

Barbara was much quicker than I would have been – her first and only question was: "Did you take them out of the package?"

"No," he replied, "It didn't say to do that on the instructions."

"Well, they just presumed you would know that the paper on the package would burn! Turn the oven off and cover the packages with a wet towel or wet cloth to put out the fire. Then take the dinners out of their packages, turn the oven back on and set it for the recommended temperature. Everything will be O.K."

It was a good thing Barbara handled the call. It would not have occurred to me that someone would not take the dinners out of the package.

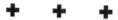

One fall evening, I finished late at the office, but had one house call to make. Hunger was motivating my hurry as I sped along 33rd Avenue S.W. The hunger pangs disappeared when I heard the siren of a motorcycle policeman. He was polite as he examined my driver's license.

"What's the reason for the big rush, Doctor?" he enquired.

"I was asked to make a house call to this address."

"My God," he said, "that's my address. What's the problem?"

"I don't really know. I was asked to see a lady who might be bleeding."

"Oh, God, my wife is about three months pregnant. Follow me," he shouted. He threw his motorcycle into gear and roared off. I did as I was instructed.

We arrived at a neat little bungalow, and rushed in to see our patient, who gave us the diagnosis: a miscarriage. This young couple were devastated. To have their first pregnancy fail in a miscarriage is a crushing experience.

Arrangements were made for her admission to hospital. No comment nor action was taken in response to my speeding. I wouldn't want to depend on that kind of co-incidence to prevent further speeding tickets.

In those days, when we worked emergency, we got to know most of the duty policemen. It was not a reason to bend the rules. One Sunday morning, driving over to the Calgary General Hospital with the children in the back seat, I came to a railway crossing and did not make a complete stop, easing through the crossing.

On the other side of the tracks, I noticed, but ignored, a motorcycle policeman. He walked over and said, "You know better than that Doctor. You did not come to a complete stop, as the law requires, before you crossed the tracks."

Our conversation was slowed when my three year old son, engrossed with the sight of the policeman's holstered revolver at his eye level, said from the back seat, "Are you going to shoot my daddy 'cause he didn't stop?"

He said, "Get out of here. You know better. I'm not going to argue with your son, now scoot!" He was understanding because he had a son the same age.

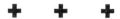

Dr. Noel Smith practiced in Calgary, a member of the C.P.R. Clinic. An Irishman of large proportions, he was loved by all, his patients, confreres and colleagues. Everyone though the world of him with good reason: he cared.

As a student in Ireland, he had formed his own dance band to put himself through university. He played the piano and saxophone superbly. As a spin off after a dull meeting of the Calgary and District Medical Society, some of us hung behind and the nucleus of the Medical Band was born.

We played for student nurses' dances at their Calgary General Hospital residence. Discipline in the band was strict: wear a tuxedo, no booze, get someone to take your calls, no leaving in the middle of the engagement and no charges for your playing. We had a great time; during intermission there was usually a skit, student nurses taking off the doctors, particularly those playing in the band. It was fun for everyone and we took our playing quite seriously, some of us even practiced between dances.

Catastrophe occurred after the first few months. The Musician's Union said we couldn't do this without hiring a stand-by band. "Smitty" used every logical argument in the book. We didn't play from music, we only had a list of tunes noting the key and the first few notes. We didn't belong to the Union (probably that was the basic problem). We were playing for student nurses at a free dance. None of these arguments made any difference. The initial band had to break up. As a gesture of our defiance, we used the money in our music pot to buy the nurses a good Hi-Fi set and gave them a collection of records.

Years later the band was revived by a retired pediatrician and drummer, Dr. John Birrell, under the name of "The Hippocratic Oath," a name later shortened to "The Oath." Life wasn't all work!

CHAPTER X
Looking for the Cure

In mid-summer, 1965, my life was unfolding smoothly until I received job offers from four separate pharmaceutical companies, each seeking a medical director. This was heady stuff, not one offer but four. The initial flattery lasted 24 hours, then reality set in. The logical approach was to go as a free agent to Toronto and make exploratory visits from there.

The Toronto company was quickly eliminated. They were also into food, candy and cosmetic manufacturing and that just wasn't for me. The second company, Wyeth in Windsor, was intriguing. The company president and I were compatible souls and I'm sure we would have made a productive team. Our problem was his inadequate budget for the position. The other two companies were in Montreal. The president of Ayerst and I met. We could have worked together. I'm not sure why they interviewed me, because they had an excellent medical director who was bilingual and about the same age as me. I recommended they get someone younger.

The last interview was with Charles E. Frosst and Company. The vice president, an Albertan, had been a "detail man" and had called on me when I was initially in practice in Calgary. His eye had been on me for some time, as it turns out. From a medical department point of view, Frosst wanted leadership.

I remember flying to Montreal for the second interview, thinking I must be crazy to give up a well established medical practice to take on a second and new career at age 45. I didn't have to. Maybe it was time for a new challenge. I know, it was somewhat selfish on my part to disrupt the family, move them out of a comfortable home, disturb their schooling and cause a complete upheaval in my wife's life. They never once complained. In retrospect, it was good for all of us.

Initially, there were a few days when I wondered what I had done. This was a different aspect of medical practice, but I still felt that I was working to improve patient care. I could now direct my energies to developing therapeutic bullets that physicians in clinical practice could use.

The function of a medical department within a pharmaceutical company is diverse and broad. A knowledge of current products is vital since all enquiries concerning use, side effects and patient medication problems are directed to that department. Past experience as a clinician makes liaison with practicing physicians easier because physicians are more apt to listen to one of their own than someone they perceive as a pure academic or a research scientist – peculiar, but true. If you have not been one of them, they don't think you can understand. An ability to clearly comprehend the problem and an ability to develop workable solutions earns a trust which rapidly spreads throughout the working medical community. In turn, this confidence creates needed feedback and gives rise to the development of new products.

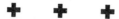

The concept of using salicylates (aspirin) as an anti-inflammatory in the treatment of arthritis is very old and the results quite good.

The gastric irritation side effects, however, can be serious and can prevent adequate dosage levels and hinder adequate treatment time. This prevented optimum use of this anti-inflammatory. We reasoned that developing a coating which allowed salicylates to pass through the stomach's acid media unchanged would eliminate this irritation. The coating was designed to break down and allow absorption in the alkali medium of the upper small bowel. This seemed a straightforward, rational idea, but there were several problems to overcome.

First, the correct coating had to be developed. A task handled by my friend, Jack Millar, head of the pharmacy research laboratory. Jack now had to develop a suitable absorbable coating material. This took many tries and indeed the selected name for the coating on Entrophen was called Polymer 37, it being the thirty-seventh compound with which he worked!

A bigger problem was coating the tablet. At that time, most tablets were coated using a technique developed in the candy industry. The coating, in liquid form, was dispersed over the tablets as they rolled in an obliquely held rotating copper drum. The coating stuck and the tablets became polished in the rolling. This technique, however, would not work for this new coating. It would not stick.

In research, the basic method of thinking is to clearly define the problem before rushing out to develop the solution. At least 80% of our effort was spent clearly defining the problem. A solution usually followed with 20% expenditure of effort.

Our basic problem was how to apply the coating to make it stick. Jack Millar and I lived at the west end of the island containing Montreal, Jack in Baie d'Urfe and me in Beaconsfield, a one-hour drive to the old Frosst plant in lower Westmount. We went together and talked shop all the way, a pleasant way to pass time.

I thought we had covered the basics of coating a tablet. You can dip it, brush it on, roll it on, spray it and electrostatically coat it. I'm sure we had covered the methods many times.

That weekend, Ruth and I were in one of the department stores when all of a sudden I noticed a vacuum cleaner display I had seen hundreds of times before. The vacuum tube was hooked into the blower end and suspended, turning and rotating in the vortex of air, were a number of colored balloons.

I said to Ruth, "Just go on and leave me here for a minute. Don't talk, just go, please, I want to watch this." She has put up with me for many years and knows when I'm crazy.

I watched that display and visualized how we could hold tablets in the vortex of air and spray a coating on, thus allowing the coating to dry evenly. I didn't know whether it would work, but it was a new approach.

When we drove to work, Jack listened while I excitedly told him about my new idea. I thought it was original, however he informed me that it wasn't. The concept went back many years, but finding the right coating materials and coating process had proven elusive. It is a long story, historically going back to June, 1959, when Dr. Dale Wurster of the Faculty of Pharmacy at the University of Wisconsin had disclosed this process of air suspension tablet coating. He dreamed this up from watching a display of fluidized ping-pong balls. However, Jack was willing to give it a try.

At Frosst, Jack Millar and Lloyd Finley initially played with a mini column consisting of a cardboard tube and a vacuum cleaner blower and this method of coating the tablets worked! Their original working column was four inches in diameter. The columns increased in size to six inches, then twelve inches and now they build many computer-controlled columns of twenty-four inches housed in separate buildings. Today, this method is used to apply coatings to the vast majority of coated tablets and the numbers of tablets are astronomical.

This was one hurdle overcome. Now we needed a marker to follow tablets through the gastro-intestinal tract and monitor their absorption. I thought this was simple. We would make up a batch of tablets, incorporating some barium sulphate as a marker. The barium would allow us to visualize the path of the tablets by x-ray. It worked fine. They showed up from one end of the gastro-intestinal tract to the other! In my mind's eye, I saw these tablets looking like a metal cleaning pad, never breaking down, never being absorbed and dropping out the bottom of the gastro-intestinal tract like a ball bearing.

When you encounter a problem, do more research. Back to the library to read, rethink, clarify and reread. My head was spinning. Morning after morning was given to the library, the afternoons to running my department and all other aspects of medicine in a pharmaceutical company.

I learned that there is a chemical bonding between barium sulphate and salicylates, our anti-inflammatory. That is why we were getting absorption of salicylates, yet the tablets didn't seem to be absorbed, didn't disappear on x-ray. We needed another marker.

Frosst being a leader in radio-active isotopes made it easy to talk to my chemistry and isotope confreres and get help. We solved the problem by using technetium as the marker.

The radio-active isotope department head was Dr. Ralph Jamieson, who had driven tourist buses for Rocky Mountain Tours in Banff about the same time I was driving for Jasper Park Lodge. It is a small world. Our paths crossed many times in the development of other products.

We now had a product which was absorbed where we had planned and the serum salicylate levels were in keeping with the oral dose and were high enough to be therapeutic. We had done the animal toxicology studies in various species. We had obtained the necessary federal department permits to allow a clinical field trial in humans. This may sound simple, but it is complex and usually takes five to eight years. Our problem was somewhat simplified because we were using a proven drug, acetylsalicylic acid – the Bayer Company's trademark name adopted by the public as Aspirin, (nicknamed ASA) – one of the basic ingredients in the Frosst line of products (i.e. 217, 222, 282, 292 – the amount of codeine being the main variable). The pharmaceutical beginnings of Frosst four generations ago were with this same basic drug, ASA, when the 200 series was developed by Mr. Charles E. Frosst, the founder.

Our initial clinical trial was carried out in the Winnipeg Rehabilitation Facility. It was not necessary to do a double-blind study. Such a study is where neither the patient nor the doctor know whether the pills contain the active ingredient. Results are recorded, then the code is broken. This is to assess whether the patient reporting improvement actually received the drug under test. This is to minimize the placebo effect, which may be as high as 10%. Our study specified serum salicylate levels at specific times throughout the 24 hours to prove correlation between the dose by mouth and the subsequently produced blood level of the drug.

As we developed and correlated our clinical data, we had a basis upon which to advise practicing physicians of side effects and anticipated results if they used this product in the treatment of their arthritic patients. This is a simplified description, but it is the essence of a clinical trial. In summary, this is the story of the development of Entrophen, twenty-five years ago.

Pharmaceutical manufacturing is clarifying a need, developing a solution, testing it, putting it through the governmental safeguards, manufacturing it in quantity, packaging, testing it to prove claims, distributing, teaching about it and continually improving the product.

It is a fascinating, competitive and intriguing business. I'm glad I was able to contribute. Frosst were looking for someone with clinical practice background to come into research and to be a part of identifying disease problems and help to develop therapeutic bullets to fire at the disease.

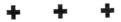

In the mid-sixties, Merck & Company, the giant U.S. pharmaceutical company, bought Charles E. Frosst & Company. Frosst was the last completely Canadian-owned pharmaceutical company doing research. The cost of research, based upon the small Canadian market and government restrictions, was becoming prohibitive. Frosst had survived not by doing basic research, but by developing improved and better products, well marketed. Making a better mousetrap, not inventing the concept of a mousetrap.

The Merck Company had a different philosophy and had worldwide markets and finances to support it. They had started many years ago as manufacturers of basic pure chemicals and dyes. Merck's philosophy in pharmaceutical research was to select a field and, in the course of doing all the research, develop pharmaceutical products. As an example, Merck did in-depth research on kidney function and the associated diseases. Using their in-depth knowledge, they developed drugs which enhance the basic kidney function. We now call that group of drugs diuretics.

Merck acquired Frosst to provide a Canadian manufacturing unit, Merck-Frosst Laboratories, with its required support facilities such as a medical department; organizationally it stands in the centre of two sales forces and their respective products on each side. The central unit manufactures products and labels them for either the Merck side or the Frosst side. This allows a greater market penetration and sales distribution of a larger number of products. Most of the basic research direction and manufacturing expertise remains at Merck's head office in Rahway, New Jersey, U.S.A.

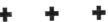

Another adventure involved anti-depressant drugs. Years ago Frosst started selling one of the early anti-depressants. The Frosst salesmen, many of whom were pharmacists, were not accustomed to calling on psychiatrists who dealt with mental illness exclusively. Psychiatrists are unique, particularly so up until the late '60s. Maybe it was because the psychiatrists had so few forms of treatment, so few drugs gave good, positive results. They still don't have many mind drugs, but the situation is improving.

In trying to teach the sales staff about depression and psychiatrists, I had to recall my experiences in practice. At that time, based on personal experience, I knew and respected one psychiatrist. More came later. Morris, it seemed to me, had only two diagnoses, the patients were nuts, or they were not nuts.

Years before, I had had a patient I had diagnosed as having Korsakoff's Psychosis, a severe mental illness. I asked Morris to see him in consultation. Morris' hospital consultation report was short and to the point: "This man is nuts. I will make the necessary arrangements to transfer him to the Mental Hospital in Ponoka." I went to Morris the next morning and said, "Thank you for seeing that patient. I know he is nuts. Do you think it is Korsakoff's Psychosis?"

Morris looked at me, pondered a moment and said, "Does it really make a difference whether the diagnosis is put in this pigeonhole or that? He is crazy. We don't have any satisfactory treatment other than confinement." Morris was a compassionate man working against tremendous odds.

This was the moment I thought I could get to the bottom of a problem that had bothered me for years. I couldn't resist the temptation to ask, "Morris, tell me, why are most of you fellows in psychiatry crazy?"

He gave me the best answer I ever heard: "At least half of the people in this specialty went into psychiatry looking for a solution to their own problems. They haven't as yet found their solutions!"

The above did not apply to Morris. He was an extremely sane man who worked hard in a sea of crazy people, some of whom were doctors.

Frosst was sending its salesmen, who had previously only sold pain killers and other medications, into this world of psychiatric problems. I had to teach them that psychiatrists could not look into their minds. Basically, psychiatrists behave like the rest of us.

I was most interested in the effectiveness and side effects of a new anti-depressant, one of the early amitriptyline group of drugs, still in the initial stages of introductory use. To this end, I had repeatedly instructed the detail men to clearly learn what problems the doctors were having. Not necessarily to answer the problems – pass that on to me – but clearly define the problem and I would follow up.

You can image my amusement one morning receiving a hand-written note from the detail man covering Sarnia. His note read: "Doctor so and so says the bloody stuff doesn't work!"

Now I had 4000 cases of initial clinical trial studies proving that the "bloody stuff" did work. So I phoned the doctor. He was amazed; no one from a pharmaceutical company had ever responded to his comments in the past. This was his red-letter day! When he learned he was talking to a doctor who had actually practiced and treated sick people, I was well accepted.

After the pleasantries, we got to the point. "Why do you say the bloody stuff doesn't work?" I asked.

"Well, the first case I tried it on was my wife," he replied, "and she said it did nothing. I could not detect any improvement. I know the treatment takes a few weeks, but she was on it for six weeks."

"There must be a reason, some explanation. Tell me your wife's past medical history, please," I said.

I learned she had surgery on her thyroid and also the surgical removal of a portion of her upper small bowel. That specific area, unfortunately, happened to be the site of absorption of the second metabolite, the active ingredient of this drug. No wonder it didn't work.

I was able to explain the mechanism of action of this product to him and why, in truth, the bloody stuff had not worked for his wife, since she had lost the portion of bowel which absorbed the drug. He was reasonable. I enquired about his training, which was good. I asked how long he had been in clinical practice and about how many cases of depression he would treat in a month. The figures were high average, so I decided to try turning his outlook on our product around.

"You have considerable clinical skills in this area. You are the type of experienced clinician I need to assess this drug at this stage of its development," I said. "I now have records on 4000 cases in which it works. That is why I am now particularly interested in cases, like your wife's, where there is a therapeutic problem. If I send you the literature and supply of samples, would you run a clinical trial for me on about a dozen cases? I know you fellows hate paperwork. I have set up a system where, by calling a special number, you can dictate your report, tell us what happened. We'll type up the report and send you a copy. You can contribute to this overall clinical trial."

He was enthusiastic and followed through with about 30 cases, all well documented and a great help.

The next day, the comptroller visited my office. He was again trying to cut expenses. His opening salvo was: "Do you know how much your long distance bill was last month?"

"I have no idea," I replied, "I use it when I need to do so."

"Well, it was almost $125," he glowered.

"Is that all? It must have been a quiet month. When I was in practice and on a lot of committees, my office long distance charges were often more than that."

Once that exchange was over, I got serious and reviewed with him how much trouble I would have been in had I tried to answer the doctor's statement about the bloody stuff not working when I had no knowledge of the patient's surgical history. As a senior company officer, I would have projected an image of company stupidity and insensitivity. Some-times you have to get down to basics. If we couldn't afford long distance follow-up calls, we should not be in business.

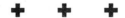

We worked with a number of drugs in preliminary stages; some needed further development. Some did not. We worked to develop a drug for the treatment of cancer of the prostate. It didn't have a name, only a number. Initially, it showed great potential. We thought we were on to something, there being no satisfactory treatment for prostate cancer. Unfortunately, the drug was unstable. We would make it and in a matter of three weeks it had changed into another compound. The initial compound seemed to be effective. The subsequent was not toxic, but it did nothing. With a shelf-life of only three weeks, it was impossible to consider manufacture and distribution. It was another blind alley, a contributor to the roller coaster of emotions in research.

At Frosst, we put time and money into developing a child-proof or safe medication container. However, there were problems. If we developed a container children could not easily open, elderly people with arthritic hands and diseases producing weak gripping muscles could not open it. A lot of bright people struggled with that one with limited success.

The best we came up with was the "Blister Pak," that frustrating pill push-through where they won't go through easily. Or the totally con-tained blister pak where you usually use scissors. They have a degree of child safety. The kids get bored before they removed enough pills to be poisoned.

There doesn't seem to be a simple answer. Children are inventive and curious. Thank goodness, because they are our future inventors. Adults frustrate easily and they didn't ask for arthritic joints and weak muscles.

One area we have to watch is making medication too attractive. If we make it look like candy and taste like candy, we are going to have tragedies. Marketing cannot be allowed to get ahead of common sense safety practices.

Alternate routes of giving medication are developing. I don't mean injection, I mean transdermal absorption, through the skin. This isn't new, just redeveloped. Initially it was female hormones, then nitroglycerine. I'm sure that is just the beginning. I can see using this route for medication where we wish a prolonged active effect, steady, rather than peaks and valleys. The first that comes to mind is aminophylline as a broncho-dila-tor, and nicotine to let the addict down slowly is presently available. As we develop new medication vehicles, we will develop alternate methods. Always safety, then convenience, not the reverse.

+ + +

I'm convinced comptrollers and computers are born without a sense of humor. I was often called to New York for several days. While there, a crisis would develop in some part of the country and I would grab a flight involving travel to several cities before I returned to Montreal.

Years earlier, when I was working for Imperial Oil Limited, the medical director explained expense accounts: "Count the amount of money you have before you leave; detail your expenses in categories of transportation, meals, hotel, taxis and tips; when you return, count what's left and the difference is your expenses. You do not include any personal purchases. You will never make any money on your expense account."

With those principles as a guide, I submitted my expense accounts. Having a professional staff who also travelled, and whose expense accounts crossed my desk, gave me a clear idea of costs in doing business. The padded expense account stood out boldly.

My expense accounts always included an item "L. and P.A." This was for an irregular sum such as $14.93 or $21.82. These items passed without question for six months. In time, the comptroller came to my office seeking an explanation of my code. He did not have such a category on the computer. Our conversation was interesting.

MR. COMPTROLLER:

"We notice a recurring item on your expense accounts, 'L. and P.A.' – what is this? We do not have such a category on the computer."

DEFENDANT (ME):

"It's very simple. Not the least bit complex. When I leave on a trip, I count the money in my pocket. When I get back, I recount the money and distribute the expenses in categories outlined on the expense account voucher.

There is usually a slight financial shortfall because I don't remember the exact tip I gave the bellhop who roomed me, nor the exact cost of a taxi, not the cost of a bouquet I used to persuade an uncooperative receptionist to let me see a doctor. The shortfall is covered in 'L. and P.A.'"

MR. COMPTROLLER:

"I still don't understand."

DEFENDANT:

"It is really simple. I thought you fellows would have figured it out by now. The symbols stand for 'Lost and Pissed Away.' It covers the financial shortfall, details of which escape my memory when rushing around the country handling emergencies."

The was a long and somewhat strained pause. Then Mr. Comptroller said, "Really, we cannot have this." He seemed very puzzled, certainly not amused. "There is no such category in the computer and we cannot balance."

"Well, what do you want me to do – falsify?" I asked him. "Do you want it in laundry or taxis or what? At least my system is honest and tells what happened."

"Possibly that's true," he replied cautiously, "but the computer is having a problem with your expense accounts. We would appreciate your clearing this matter up so we can balance!"

I had messed with the precious system. Thereafter my shortfall went into the taxi category. I used many taxis.

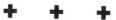

Charles E. Frosst & Co. was involved in the manufacture and sale of many products overseas. With two other companies, we shared manufacturing facilities in Beirut, Lebanon and Bogota, Columbia. Sales were in Great Britain, with some in the East and throughout the Caribbean. Dr. Fernando Ruggeri was the overseas medical director, theoretically on my staff although I let him work on his own. We sometimes travelled together, especially to New York. Since we were in adjacent rooms, it quickly became apparent to me that he didn't drink. His expense accounts, however, didn't support this theory. He picked up more than his share of bar chits.

Fernando was Italian, his father an international architect, their home Genoa, where Fernando grew up. He spoke English with a slight British accent, having trained in the U.K. Of the five medical men in the department, we two had practiced medicine and treated sick people. The others were researchers.

We arrived in New York late one afternoon and I suggested we have a Scotch before supper. He confessed he didn't drink. While practicing in Gibraltar, he explained, he had suffered a severe attack of viral hepatitis and thought it wise not to further insult his liver by asking it to work harder detoxifying alcohol. I asked him how he handled this with the amount of entertaining he was doing; I knew it was substantial, because I signed his expense reports. He gave a very clear and enlightened explanation. No one makes you drink. They don't force your jaws open and pour it down. When he was ordering drinks, he would order a gin and tonic and three twists of lime, then quietly ask them to hold the gin. Now I knew why he took the initiative in ordering drinks.

"What do you do when someone gives you a drink?" I asked.

"Again," he said, "no one forces your jaw open and pours it in. You carry it around and deposit bits of it in the potted palms."

He taught me many tricks used in teaching alcoholics a practical approach to handling their problem. Fernando was not an alcoholic, just a very intelligent man who thought for himself and made his own decisions. He is now retired, but I'm sure he is still thinking and solving problems.

The medical department always enjoyed his return from a foreign trip. If something unusual happened to him, and it usually did, his telling of it was masterful.

During a trip to our plant in South America – Bogota, Columbia – he was met by the plant superintendent and greeted in English. That was the language used for the next two days, during which Dr. Ruggeri was inspecting the plant and discussing business and medical proposals. During this period, people came to the superintendent with problems and messages. The business language of the plant was Spanish. The superintendent must not have done his homework on Dr. Ruggeri, whose wife was Spanish, a language he spoke well. He was also, obviously, fluent in English, Italian, French and German.

The superintendent often gave messages and instructions like "No, we don't want him to see that," and there were snide remarks in Spanish which Dr. Ruggeri was not supposed to understand.

At the conclusion of his trip, when the superintendent was seeing him off and wishing him well, Dr. Ruggeri could not resist thanking him for his hospitality in perfect Spanish. Looking out the plane window, Dr. Ruggeri recalled, "This chap's jaw was still on the ground in amazement." The perfect squelch!

Dr. Ruggeri was good for me, we stimulated each other's minds. Later, when involved with the cancer clinics, I tried to persuade him to join me in Edmonton and return to clinical medicine. He had already been offered an important European job with Merck and regretfully declined my offer.

CHAPTER XI

Caring and Cancer

On a routine trip West, during the summer of 1967, I stopped to see the Minister of Health of Alberta. Dr. J. Donovan Ross, a medical practitioner, was known to me through my work with the Alberta College of Physicians and Surgeons and the Alberta College of Family Practice. I anticipated this would be a quick social call. His secretary was pleased to see me, remarking, "We have been looking all over for you."

"Well, I don't know why you couldn't find me, my office in Montreal knows my itinerary and my secretary knows my whereabouts," I replied.

Apparently, my personal secretary was off sick and the remaining staff were unsure of the geography. They only knew I was "Out West." They had all been born and raised in Eastern Canada and the West created mental images of growing wheat, raising cattle and uncertain visions of oil wells.

I soon found out why Dr. Ross had been looking for me; he wanted me to leave Charles E. Frosst and Company and return to Alberta to assist him in building, staffing and operating the Dr. W.W. Cross Cancer Hospital in Edmonton, and subsequently to reorganize and operate all the cancer clinics in the province of Alberta. The official position was Executive Medical Director for the Provincial Cancer Hospital Board. I would be responsible for the Cancer Clinics and Cancer Treatment Facilities for the Province of Alberta. This was a newly created position and a newly created board. The responsibilities were awesome, yet exciting.

The Cancer Clinics in Edmonton, Calgary and Lethbridge had grown since their creation in the late '40s. Their history was a story of chronic shortages in space, staff, funding and equipment, all fuelled by the pressure of increasingly large case loads and requests for patient care.

Dr. Ross' request was not what I had expected in my routine social call. He wanted me to begin immediately. I felt I should give Frosst adequate notice and assist them in finding a replacement. We settled on me giving three months' notice.

My time as executive medical director of Frosst had been an interesting and challenging experience. Returning to research and learning the development of new drugs and products from the conceptual idea to the final product on the market and dealing with all the hurdles along the line, was educational in all aspects of management. I was not sorry I had followed the intriguing side trip; now it was time to return to clinical medicine.

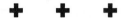

Our move west was timed to allow John and Nancy to start school in September. I followed in October. There were no suitable houses to purchase or rent, so we lived in the Riviera Hotel for some months while we built a house. They were good to us. We were moved into a corner section of rooms, allowing each of the children to have a desk and their own bathroom. We had a separate bed and bath unit. They allowed the children to practice their musical instruments, trumpet and clarinet, in the ballroom early each morning. They fed the children breakfast with immediate service in the coffee shop, knowing they had to get to school, always loading John's plate with teenage-sized servings. We appreciated their special attention.

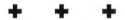

The Dr. W.W. Cross Cancer Hospital was named after a previous Alberta Minister of Health. The building of this Specialty hospital was an interesting, busy experience, accomplished with tremendous help, from an outstanding staff, gathered from around the world.

We developed innovative ideas, escalators to move ambulatory patients to radiation therapy; ward microwave ovens to supply off-hour meals; and silent independent rooms for seriously ill patients in which they controlled the bed contours and lighting. The busy Chapel contained interchangeable symbols, a Star of David and a Christian Cross. This oasis of calm was in constant use by patients and relatives and some doctors.

We constructed an outpatients' department which was bright, full of color and light, accented with multiple blooming plants and flowers. Patient morale was boosted. The department design allowed smooth patient flow without a feeling of confusion or pressure.

When we thought we had everything in place, but before we admitted any patients, we had a dry run. Over a long weekend, we admitted about twenty staff members, wrote false histories and attached appropriate diagnoses, wrote appropriate orders, medication and radiation therapy treatments. This was done in all seriousness. We took the patients to therapy by stretcher, put them under machines, set the control and kept them there for the correct time. The only thing we didn't do was turn the machines on. Everything else was done as if they were receiving treatment. We fed them, bathed them, put them in pyjamas, the full routine. Our medication orders were delivered as if it were actual medication. In reality, we used Smarties, color-coded for each medication prescribed.

We admitted four children of different ages, offspring of staff members. We had patients booked and taken to the surgical suite for mock surgery. We tried as much as possible to recreate the actual operation of the hospital. We kept notes of everything. We then had a three-day meeting to assess the deficiencies and create solutions.

We then opened the hospital for real patients. Our trial run had paid dividends. We encountered no serious problem for which we had not already created a solution. The dry run saved worries and possible tragedies. In fact, the operation ran so smoothly, we wondered what we had overlooked. Even as time passed, nothing showed up. For this I gave thanks to a dedicated and knowledgeable staff, all of whom worked hard to achieve success.

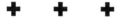

During a time of new staff training, shortly after opening the Dr. W. W. Cross Cancer Hospital, several radon seeds were temporarily lost. We wondered if they had been inadvertently thrown into the garbage and subsequently went down the sewer. This produced an initial feeling of panic and resulted in a meticulous, well-organized search.

Radon seeds or needles are fine hollow tubes of a gold amalgam which contain radon gas as a source of radiation. These are used in the treatment of solid tumors, such as cancer of the cervix. This source of radiation has an extremely long life. When not in use, they are stored in lead-lined safes to protect personnel. To have these fine needles rocketing down the sewer, being caught up by chance, who knows where, might expose the populace to unneeded and unsafe radiation. We had to find them, that very night!

The handling and safe storage of this source of radiation is the responsibility of the physicists on staff at the hospital. We searched everywhere within the building, our scientific "sniffer" a geiger counter. These counters register radiation by producing a clicking sound, the closer the source of radiation, the more rapid and insistent the clicking.

Throughout the building we searched and failed. We looked everywhere, in every garbage container, every cupboard. Where next? The only logical answer was the sewers. Night was approaching, although it makes little difference from the inside of a sewer. A thorough search was the only answer and we proceeded step by slippery, smelly step, constantly listening for an outburst of clicks from our counters. By now, we were well within the open draining main sewer conduits. I won't describe the contents of raw sewage; your imagination can supply the details, and even so, it is probably incomplete. After several hours in this unique environment, we were successful. A great burst of clicking, some probing with tongs and we retrieved our elusive radon needles. The were clinging together in a wad of gauze. Our mission was completed and no harm had ensued. We all had showers and then were clean enough to go home for a late-night supper.

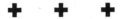

We had a few outpatients with artificial noses and ears attending the Dr. W.W. Cross Cancer Institution. It comes as a surprise to most people that these patients need a set of summertime ears or noses and a wintertime set. The color of the two sets differs.

It is almost impossible to construct acceptable artificial noses or ears throught the science of plastic surgery. More satisfactory results are achieved by custom building them from synthetic materials which can be color-shaded and texture designed. We usually had this done through the dental faculty at the university. It was a chance for some of the more talented students to earn extra money and it provided a much better one-on-one service for our patients, the alternative being mail-service from Toronto.

I had a 74-year old outpatient who had lost her entire nose due to the ravages of squamous cell carcinoma. She wore a custom-built external nose, hung from the frame of her spectacles. She was a farm lady, outside for long periods during the summer.

From the Minister of Health, I had requisitioned a summer nose. This request was vehemently denied, with a side note that said it was a "silly request." That got my dander up. The minister and I were not sympatico. He was a non-medically trained person, in reality a petroleum engineer, parachuted into the portfolio for political reasons. Maybe he had been improperly advised by one of his deputies.

I was determined to get this patient the nose she required. Her deformity was bad enough without bringing it to everyone's attention by having five shades lighter in the centre of her face. She was an independent, feisty lady, just the personality I needed for my scheme.

With her cooperation, I was sure we could get the prosthesis she needed. I explained the physical layout of the minister's office and told her she would be going through a double set of doors before she came face to face with the minister behind his imposing desk. I would make an appointment for her and as she stood before his desk, she could introduce herself and remind him she had come to explain why she needed a different colored nose for the summer. She would then take off her glasses, and with them her nose.

This creates a most startling sight. There is no nose, just an open cavity with mucous membrane-covered turbinate bones, a deep, black hole. I had warned her that he was not a medical man and that he might gag. He did.

We received our requisitioned summer nose and we sent our thank-you letters.

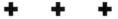

As the hospital settled into smooth operation, and as our staff requirements were gradually filled, the provincial needs of the Cancer Hospital Board shifted to the top of our priority list. Cancer clinics were developed in Medicine Hat and Red Deer, as well as a travelling clinic established into the north of the province. This acted as the precursor to a permanent clinic in Peace River. We had outgrown the Holy Cross Hospital site in Calgary. Initial planning involved the Colonel Belcher Hospital, ideal because of its central location and excellent access to public transportation facilities. Unfortunately, it was not available for political reasons and because the cost of renovation was prohibitively high. Ultimately, a separate facility was built adjacent to the Foothills Hospital. The Tom Baker Cancer Centre was named after the initial chairman of the Provincial Cancer Hospitals Board.

CHAPTER XII

Odds and Ends

My commitment to the Provincial Cancer Hospital Board really ended when I completed the tasks I had promised Dr. J. Donavan Ross I would do. I missed clinical practice. I knew in my heart I was not a civil servant and, further, government service had lost its appeal. Ruth and I missed Calgary, so we went back.

I went to the hospitals to renew medical acquaintances and encountered Dr. Vernon Fanning. He had been one of my interns many years earlier at the Calgary General Hospital.

"What are you doing with yourself these days?" he asked.

"I'm planning on returning to practice," I replied. "I'm looking for a good location and an office. It's too crowded and there's no parking around my old location, the Academy Building."

Jokingly, he said, "Do you still know how to run a practice? Why don't you come down to the Willow Park Clinic and run my office for the afternoon to get your hand back in. I'll play golf."

Without really thinking, I said, "You're on!"

He played golf and I saw fifty patients, a heavy load for an afternoon. I wasn't out of there until seven o'clock that evening and Vern had a great round of golf.

Shortly thereafter, I was invited to join the group in the Willow Park Clinic, consisting of partners and salaried doctors in both the Acadia-Fairview Clinic and Willow Park Clinic. This was the initial step in re-establishing myself in family practice.

On my first holiday weekend, working at the Willow Park Clinic for Dr. Fanning, I was surprised to get a call from the Calgary Zoo. I learned that Dr. Fanning had friends at the zoo and they often called with veterinary-medical problems. This was before the zoo had their veterinary staff. The call involved developing an infant feeding formula for a rejected newborn chimp. For reasons unknown to me, the mother chimpanzee had rejected her offspring and refused to breast feed him. Logic told me newborns are newborns. We worked out an infant formula based on the young chimp's weight. The keeper and his wife adopted the newborn chimp and he lived with them for six months until big enough to stand a chance of fending for himself.

Another time I got a call about a giraffe. They thought it had a sore throat. How does one look down a giraffe's throat? Obviously, the first requirement was a ladder or a fork lift. Joking aside, giraffes are similar to people, just bigger, and the drug doses are bigger, in keeping with their weight. Taking the animal's history is a bit more difficult. You depend on what the keepers have observed in the animal's behavior. The zoo kept me on my toes.

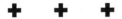

I had been at the Willow Park Clinic for about three months when Vern Fanning approached me and said, "We partners own land in Bonavista, the next district south, and ultimately we would like to build another clinic there. We wonder if you would consider taking space in the shopping center and establishing an office? If it is successful, we will consider building a clinic on the land we own."

This looked like a marvellous opportunity to me. I could start there, do things my own way and the other two clinics would be back-up. We lived in the Bonavista district, so we were already a part of that community.

This project was started in late 1970 and prospered. We were busy from the very first day. Surprisingly, a lot of my old patients from five years past returned. We had some great reunions. The little children were now big, some even in university.

The space we occupied was across the shopping mall from the drug store, originally Cunningham's, now Shoppers Drug Mart. Dr. George Sanderson, a dentist and Dr. Garth Mann, an optometrist, started their practices across the mall about the same time.

We became sufficiently busy, that at the end of one year Dr. Bill Beiber joined me and we continued to build the practice. The ultimate plan was to construct a family practice clinic on our land north of the Inn on Lake Bonavista.

This came to pass with some difficulty. We had to overcome initial opposition in the community, caused by a simple misunderstanding. Rumors spread suggesting that ambulances would be rushing to the clinic at all hours of the day and night. Once the community understood our intentions, we received full cooperation. We moved in the fall of 1974. There were multiple offices, family physicians, psychologists, an x-ray, laboratory and physiotherapy. Initially we tried to incorporate the Well Baby Clinics and the District Public Health Facility, but this was too progressive for the government. The availability of psychologists was great in clarifying and treating emotional problems.

We created a well-rounded, balanced family practice facility for the community, who appreciated it by coming as patients.

Originally, each medical office was run full-time as a single doctor's office. With the passage of time and an increased number of female medical practitioners, many of whom are handling the increased responsibility of a family, medical practices are shared. Two practitioners handle a single practice by splitting the office responsibilities. I believe this custom will gradually increase, since often both parents are working outside the home.

Over the past twenty years, the medical personnel have changed. Doctors have retired or gone to other locations or responsibilities. In addition, the working relationships have changed. We abandoned the partnership format some years ago; the age spread of the group was too great, the cost of buying in too expensive and the end-point business ambitions of the younger members were short term. They did not want to be tied to long term financial commitments, which happens when a group constructs a clinic building.

The result was a dissolution of the partnership and the formation of a loose working relationship within the clinic. The buildings were sold, as well as the labs and x-ray. This has eliminated group businesses and is more acceptable to the present members; in any case, the previous group was getting too large to administer efficiently.

Looking back, it is interesting to have lived through all methods of practice: solo, company employee, government employee, hired salaried physician, large partnership and lastly, a return to being a solo practitioner within a group. Each has had its pluses and minuses.

As I think back, interesting cases arise in my memory.

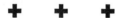

A patient phoned my nurse to enquire – could Dr. Ibberson remove an earring from her mother's ear and how much would this cost, since she was visiting from Scotland and did not have Alberta Health Care coverage?

My nurse Marie reassured her that I could probably solve such a problem and the charge would be in keeping with the time required.

In due course, this delightful Scottish grandmother appeared with an earring lodged firmly in her right ear lobe.

We started with surgical forceps. No results. Local anaesthetic was injected into the ear lobe and we got down to serious work with needle nose pliers and side cutters, instruments usually reserved for fish hook injuries. After using more strength than surgical technique, the earring was removed. The earring post was of 22K gold and had become bent resulting in a hook on the end.

We straightened the post. In a Glasgow accent, she enquired, "How much is your fee, Doctor?"

She looked like she had a sense of humor, so I said, "I don't believe you have brought sufficient funds on your trip to this country to cover my fee." After a pause, I added, "There will be no charge, it will be my contribution to your first Canadian trip." She chuckled and thanked me.

We left the examining room and a red headed, freckled, five year old burst from the reception room. After pulling my pant leg, he queried, "Did you have to unscrew Grandma's ear right off her head, to get the earring out?"

After appropriate laughter, I told Grandma "I was just paid my fee. I hope you have a nice stay in Canada."

Little people have always made my day.

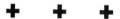

In the middle of a busy afternoon, as I moved from one examining room to the next, I noticed my nurse assisting a middle aged man into an examining room. He was in obvious discomfort – no, he was in pain. What caught my attention was his shuffle, and he had three neck ties knotted together, rope-wise, running across one shoulder and under his groin to support a small pillow.

From this, I guessed the diagnosis – prolapsed haemorrhoids. Subsequent examination confirmed my suspected diagnosis. He had severely prolapsed and several thrombosed haemorrhoids. The technical details of the therapeutic measures are found in major surgical textbooks. With the judicious and skillful use of injected local anaesthetic and the surgical removal of clots from the thrombosed haemorrhoids, he experienced miraculous relief.

Now, having granted the patient a reprieve, was the time to learn the rest of his medical history. An aerial photographer by trade, he had been working in the Lethbridge district when he first started having problems. He had attended my old friend Dr. Frank Christie for temporary relief. He knew his next assignment was Calgary, so he enquired from Dr. Frank Christie who he could see if his problem recurred. Dr. Frank knew they would.

From the patient's own mouth came Dr. Christie's answer. "There is an idiot friend of mine practicing in the south part of Calgary. He is in the Bonavista Clinic, I think he started it. I have know him for many years, he took good care of an old aunt of mine, he says he knows something about practicing medicine, I think maybe he does. See him if you are in trouble."

What a great recommendation for a referral. It does sound exactly like Frank Christie, short and to the point.

Our haemorrhoid friend was in trouble. We got him over the immediate emergency and then carried out a planned surgical repair.

He was so grateful, as a gift he brought a bottle of Scotch whiskey when he came for his final post operative examination.

Now that is gratitude! Since he was the last patient of the day, we tested its purity.

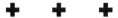

Recently, the nurse of one of my female confreres came flying into my office to ask, "Do you have any special instruments for removing a peanut from a child's nose?"

"Not really," I answered. "You don't need special surgical instruments, you make what you need using a paper clip."

Not surprisingly, she didn't believe me. Maybe I had been too abrupt, so I said, "I have a special light that I use to visualize vocal cords and it is good to illuminate the nose and ear. You really do make up what you need from paper clips – do you need any help?"

As I walked down the hall to their office, I took a paper clip, a pair of needle nosed pliers (usually used to remove fish hooks) and my special light.

In my confrere's office was red headed three year old, all male. When I asked him why he put a peanut in his nose, he shrugged and did not answer. It was a stupid question, I should have know better; I presume he put it there, as all boys do, to see where it would go. Well, it went well back behind the inferior turbinate bone just in front of his soft palate. Just ready to drop into his windpipe and obstruct his breathing.

He wasn't concerned, however, I was. It could fall into the back of his throat and in the excitement be inhaled into his windpipe and thence into his lung. Peanuts and lungs do not live well together. A minor inconvenience then becomes a major emergency, requiring immediate surgical intervention.

Grasping the peanut with forceps usually results in failure and the peanut is pushed further back or crushed, which is worse since peanut particles are inhaled and you cannot flush out the lungs!

The are two tricks: explanation and a custom made tool. I am always amazed at what you can do to children, if you give them a complete explanation and handle them with complete honesty. While I was straightening the paper clip and forming a tiny looped hook at one end, making a right-angled handle at the other end, I tried to explain in detail to my red-headed friend exactly what we were going to do.

I said, "It will take two of us to do this job. You have to keep your head quite still. I'll ask the nurse to help you hold it still. I have to slip this special tool into your nose. It will tickle but it won't hurt. Once we are past the peanut, then we turn the tool and flip out the peanut. That might hurt for just a second, but don't turn your head – then it's all over.

We did just that, one flip and I caught the peanut.

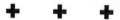

Some years ago I examined a middle aged female patient who complained of a skin rash. She told me she had consulted two younger practitioners earlier, without being given a diagnosis. Rather than blurt out the diagnosis, I persisted in learning her medical history. I told her I knew the diagnosis based on cases I had seen during the war. She had the typical rash of secondary syphilis.

On further questioning, she admitted to having been a Madam of a house of easy morals many years before. She did not recall any symptoms of primary syphilis, which is not unusual in females. She was now in the secondary phase of this contagious disease.

She then dropped a second pearl of wisdom, as she informed me that three of her nieces worked for Alberta Health Care in the main records and accounts office. This knowledge gave me cause for alarm, since the diagnosis must be stated on the billing slip you submit to Alberta Health Care to collect your fee. With not one niece, but three working there, my chances of the account slipping through unnoticed diminished considerably. What was I to do? On the one hand, I thought I was particularly astute to have made the diagnosis and proven it with a positive blood test; on the other hand, I didn't wish to initiate a family scandal. I thought about it for several days, then asked my staff to submit the billing slip with the diagnosis: a specific dermatitis caused by a spirochaetal infection. If the nieces were smart enough to figure out the pathological terminology, they were entitled to know their Aunt's diagnosis.

The account went through routinely, maybe they didn't see it, maybe they were discreet. With adequate penicillin therapy, we cured the infection.

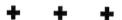

One day, immediately preceding the Calgary Olympic Games, I walked into an examining room and met a lady I hadn't seen in many years. Her children had grown, gone through university and she had moved to another part of the city and been healthy.

"Well hello, what brings you in to see me after all these years?"

"My friends think I need to see a psychiatrist, my husband wonders."

"Knowing you as I do, and having cared for you through two pregnancies years ago, I find it hard to believe that you need a psychiatric consultation. Maybe you should tell me your story."

She worked for the Olympic organization in a senior secretarial position, near the top. I purposely did not learn for which official. She was meticulously dressed, smartly turned out. This tended to rule out the diagnosis of a deep depression. She seemed genuinely distraught, and yet this was a woman I knew to be emotionally stable. I recalled her husband was an engineer and they seemed to have a loving, solid marriage. Amazing what your mind can recall about a patient's past history in an instant. Usually I can't recall a patient's name, but I can easily remember important detailed past history and medications tolerated.

As her history unfolded, it was obvious the media had been writing and saying negatively critical things about the Olympic organization. When you are in the public eye, you are fair game for criticism in this day of the negative approach. It seemed she was starting to believe all these adverse written and spoken words.

After exploring her anxieties in detail, it was obvious she did not need a psychiatric consultation. She did not have a mental illness. She had an exaggerated anxiety.

With a grin, I said to her, "The last person you need to see is a psychiatrist. We don't want to reinforce this anxiety."

"Hmm, let me see, the solution to your problem is two-fold. The first part is easy, the second a little tricky and involves the use of street talk. Your husband being an engineer and having raised sons, I'm sure you have heard this language before."

"First, we quit reading and listening, ignore what the media are writing or saying. They are not responsible for putting on the Games, they criticize and generate copy and develop hype. All necessary pre-motivational activities for the public."

"The second part of the solution is a bit more difficult to explain. You are a cultured Lady and I don't wish to offend you, but you and I have been through a lot together in the past and I am going to presume on that friendship. The second part of the treatment involves a basic fundamental principal of physics, WATER RUNS DOWN HILL. You rise above these problems and these small minded people, so you can – Piss on Them. My apologies for the language but the verb urinate does not carry the same clout."

She started to laugh. She laughed so hard her mascara ran down her cheeks. She blotted. It smeared. She tried to talk, only giggles came. She made a supreme effort to gain control and almost succeeded, then dissolved into a spasm of belly shaking laughter. Finally she blurted out:

"I knew you would understand."

Then she had the giggles again. As she regained her composure, she continued.

"My husband thinks I have slipped over the brink. He will understand your language and explanation, as do I. Don't you remember, I grew up with three older brothers and have two sons. I may try to be a Lady, but I'm not deaf."

Then she had a fresh attack of giggles, wiped her nose and tried to repair her smeared mascara.

"I love your explanation and solution!"

The word solution set her off again, but gradually she was gaining the upper hand. I wondered what the patients waiting in the reception room would think of this crying, giggling, middle aged Mom? What would they think of me? Of my image...forget it. I didn't care to have an image, everyone knew I was a nut.

I didn't see her again in my office, but I did ask her to please call me in a week to report her progress.

She called and I asked, "How are you doing? Are you coping?"

"Oh yes, well, thank you." She started to giggle but checked it.

"I have had a sign made, to sit on my desk. Initially I typed it, later I had a proper sign printed."

Oh, my gosh, I thought, surely she didn't have them print up a big sign with my punch line.

With trepidation, I whispered, "What does the sign say?"

"Not what you imagine; sometimes I think you are really bad, at least naughty."

She was going to keep me dangling, probably because I made her mascara streak.

"It just says, WATER RUNS DOWN HILL. That's enough. Some people ask, but that's enough. You have restored my sanity. Thank you for understanding."

She did not need follow up. We all know the Games went off superbly. When in doubt remember, WATER RUNS DOWN HILL.

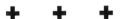

Recently, I was a patient. Doctors do get sick, kidney stones again. As my loving wife Ruth says, "Some fellows have rocks in their head, yours, dear, have always been in your kidneys." Recovering from another surgical approach to remove the offending stones from the left kidney, I felt pretty perky on my third post operative day. The evening-shift nurse, whom I have know for some years, came in to get me settled for the night and said, "Is there anything else I can do for you, to make you comfortable?"

I just could not resist such an opening, and asked, "Don't I get a good-night kiss?"

She wasn't put off, she didn't misunderstand. She said, "We are pretty busy on the floor tonight, I'll see what I can do about it."

I should have known I was in trouble; after all, I have been around nurses most of my life.

About twenty minutes later, she quietly entered my room, holding a 10cc syringe with a four inch long spinal needle attached, and cooed, "Where would you like your good-night kiss?"

Never underestimate the imagination these ladies possess. I deserved it and should have known better.

I hope I made it up to them with chocolates and flowers. They earned a reward for professional and imaginative nursing. They are a group of special ladies.

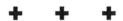

Years ago, when I hired my nurse, Marie, I was looking for a mature, experienced nurse whose background reflected experience in country hospitals. That is exactly what I got, plus a lady of great efficiency, a remarkable sense of humor and someone the patients loved. She had that magic touch of being able to handle every type of patient and every salesman's personality, and keep the ship of practice management on an even keel. Of course she handled me, too, that was an additional plus.

Every well-run office has someone who handles the boss. I was fortunate.

During our initial interview, I asked if she could type, since I prefer to dictate my office charts. She replied in the affirmative, then proceeded to learn how to type. We meshed from day one.

As we got busier, we needed a half-time secretary. Since these ladies would be sharing the same office, it was logical that Marie serve on the interview team. Her judgment has always been excellent, as was indicated when Jeane joined our team. What a joy to work with superb people who have a sense of humor. I was truly blessed.

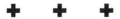

From 1950 to almost 1990, Dr. James R. Francis and I worked together. We developed a subconscious surgical thinking sense whereby we knew what the other was thinking or could anticipate the other's thoughts. We worked as a team. When we started our practices, General Surgery covered a wide field, not as restricted as it is today. He had trained in Toronto, as an early member of the Gallie course; I had trained in Vancouver.

One morning, when working at the Rockyview Hospital, the operating room nurses had set up two tables of sterile instruments for our case. Jim took one look at this impressive display and said, "The hospitals in which Ibberson and I trained could not afford this many instruments; we don't know how to use that many. Just give us this and that on a separate table. Then we won't soil the others and you won't have to rewash them. If you give us all those instruments, we will get confused."

Jim was a clear thinker, who knew his anatomy. He did not cut without having a clear plan and backup plan. In all the years we worked together, I never saw him lose his temper. When angry or upset, he spoke clearly, slowly and was definite in his instructions and commands. There could have been no doubt in anyone's mind what he wanted.

We used to say the operating nurses could always tell how things were going, depending on the side chatter. If things were going well, there was lots of chatter, if we were in difficulty, there was deep silence.

Jim was an excellent diagnostician; he would repeat his history-taking process until he uncovered every aspect of the patient's problem. When involved in a consultation between us, we would argue until we both felt satisfied that we had uncovered and understood every facet of the problem. Clinicians of this calibre are easy to work with. His father and brother had similar characteristics.

Jim died suddenly early in 1990, I'm sorry to say. He is missed by all who knew him.

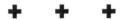

As my seventieth birthday approached I proceeded with plans to retire – I didn't want to stay on too long and fossilize. I had a young, well-trained family physician, Dr. Jim Thorne, who had shared my office for five years preparing to tend to the patients.

My most capable nurse, Mrs. Marie Hill, unknown to me, had meticulously planned a retirement dinner and dance at a nearby hotel. I could not believe the number of patients, confreres, friends and relatives who attended. Marie had arranged for messages from the Prime Minister, the Premier, the Mayor and District Alderman. The Regional MLA, Bill Payne, and his wife were also in attendance.

During the evening, humorous speeches were made by my friend, Dr. Jim Francis, and Dr. Ernest Bensler, who was President of the Bonavista Clinic Association.

The proceedings culminated with the presentation of a beautiful Longines wrist watch with the inscription "From your friends, colleagues and patients – Dr. J.R. Ibberson, 31 July 1989."

With humble pride and gratitude, I wear this watch on festive occasions.

What a grand way to end the working portion of a life privileged to serve patients and to follow my scientific interests.

CHAPTER XIII

Epilogue

The twilight of my life having commenced, after forty-five years of carrying a little black bag, allows me the luxury of reflection. I was fortunate to practice medicine in that "golden age" when many specialties were born, antibiotics were discovered and undreamed-of diagnostic methods pioneered. Major diseases fell to the onslaught of specific cure or prevention.

The generations of physicians preceding my era struggled with fatal infections, such as tuberculosis, typhoid, scarlet fever, etc. Their therapeutic tools were often limited to general supportive measures. Today we can be precise, specific and effective. The greatest good for the most people has probably been in the field of Public Health. This is based on precise laboratory work to provide a clear understanding of specific diseases. An example is Poliomyelitis, once feared, now preventable by immunization.

Before the days of medicare, we were allowed the luxury of knowing our patients well and following them in some cases from birth to death. Patients knew at first hand the cost of the services provided, since the doctor discussed his fee with each patient. The patient could request further explanation, express their gratitude or register complaints. This was the original and most effective quality control mechanism, the satisfying one-on-one method of medical practice.

Third party payers, a part of health plans and insurance coverage, introduce an impersonal bureaucratic buffer screen which replaces the personal touch. Life always involves trade-offs; there is no free lunch.

There are still many baffling diseases beyond our understanding. The public would select cancer, with some justification, but we have made great progress in understanding the basic mechanism of this disease. I would select the field of mental and emotional disease, an outstanding example being schizophrenia. There are many others in the neurological field, diseases such as multiple sclerosis. Scientists will persist in seeking more knowledge from which will come prevention or cure.

When one speculates on new ideas and developments at the cutting edge of medicine, one wishes for a return of youth. Today's young doctors anticipate the future as we did years ago, when even our imaginations were inadequate to match the speed of developments. I know today's doctors will be in a similar position when they carry a little black bag.

After five years of retirement, I have learned new skills. But I still miss the people and children, as patients.

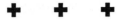